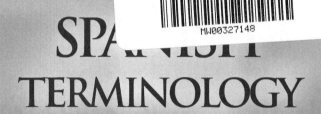

SPANISH
TERMINOLOGY
for the
EYECARE TEAM

TERMINOLOGÍA
EN ESPAÑOL
para el
EQUIPO DE CUIDADO
OCULAR

SPANISH TERMINOLOGY

for the

EYECARE TEAM

TERMINOLOGÍA EN ESPAÑOL

para el

EQUIPO DE CUIDADO OCULAR

Brian Chou, OD, FAAO
San Diego, California

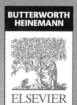

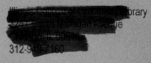

BUTTERWORTH
HEINEMANN
ELSEVIER

11830 Westline Industrial Drive
St. Louis, Missouri 63146

SPANISH TERMINOLOGY FOR   ISBN-13: 978-0-7506-7562-8
THE EYECARE TEAM   ISBN-10: 0-7506-7562-4
Copyright © 2006, Elsevier Inc.

Notice

Some material previously published, Practical Spanish in Eyecare, © 2001
Elsevier Inc.

ISBN-13: 978-0-7506-7562-8
ISBN-10: 0-7506-7562-4

Acquisitions Editor: Kathy Falk
Senior Developmental Editor: Christie Hart
Publishing Services Manager: Julie Eddy
Project Manager: Kelly E.M. Steinmann
Book Designer: Bill Drone

Printed in the United States of America
Last digit is the print number: 9 8 7 6 5

Contents

Chapter 17
Binocular Indirect Ophthalmoscopy, 52

Chapter 18
Special Ophthalmic Procedures, 54

Chapter 19
Ophthalmic Dispensary, 59

Chapter 20
Working with Children, 70

Chapter 21
Basic Explanations, 74

Chapter 22
Explanations for Specific Conditions, 91

Chapter 23
Office Administration, 101

Preface

Spanish Terminology for the Eyecare Team was designed for those committed eyecare providers desiring to improve their exam-room Spanish. Optometrists, ophthalmologists, and their ancillary staff should find it useful. Despite an oversupply of eyecare in some areas, the eye-related needs of Spanish-speakers remain largely underserved. This book is dedicated to the visual welfare of those patients, as well as the practitioners who serve them.

WHAT YOU CAN EXPECT

With a rudimentary understanding of Spanish grammar and pronunciation, this book should help you formulate explanations, instructions, and questions in Spanish. Realize, however, that any language has substantial variation in how it is spoken. Fully comprehending the responses from your patients comes through extensive practice. There is no substitute for a regimented course of listening, speaking, reading, and writing. No book by itself can provide you with all the facets of mastering a language. With that awareness, I created this book as a learning adjunct.

WHY THIS BOOK?

Perhaps the greatest strength of this book is that it was *not* authored by someone fluent in Spanish. I struggle with the language. This probably fits your own description. When I was learning to perform an exam in Spanish, I ran into recurring situations that existing literature did not address. In essence, this guide was born out of frustration. I compiled the situations in which I wished I knew what to say in Spanish. Before I knew it, the compilation became the precursor to the book you are holding.

HISTORY OF THIS BOOK

The first edition of this book, *Practical Spanish in Eyecare*, reflected my own clinical experience caring for Spanish-speaking patients. I started working on the book, unknowingly at the time, while providing charitable eyecare on various humanitarian trips. Most of the Spanish-speaking patients that I saw were poor, with little to no healthcare.

For many, my eye exam was their very first. I observed a high incidence of ocular disease. Pterygia, diabetic retinopathy, cataracts, and glaucoma were common and often in advanced stages. Consistent with these observations, the first edition did not go into detail on "elective" treatments, such as contact lenses and refractive surgery. For many of my patients, glasses would have been enough of a financial burden. Certainly, each practitioner's patient base has unique demographics, which may or may not parallel my own clinical exposure.

This second edition expands beyond the survival-level Spanish, so that the user has more than enough to make it through a basic eye examination. Besides covering contact lenses and refractive surgery in greater detail, you will find additional descriptions on common eye conditions and material to help your front staff interact with Spanish-speaking patients. I am most excited by the inclusion of a CD-ROM, which will help you learn pronunciation. You can even use the CD-ROM in conjunction with an exam-room computer to play selected sentences to your patient.

GOOD CASE HISTORY: A MIX OF QUESTIONS

As you'll see, several patient questions have binary answers (e.g., "yes" or "no," "right" or "left") or at least relatively limited answers. They can be very useful, especially to those new to Spanish, because the possible answers tend to have less variation. Although it is reassuring to ask these questions, clinicians should not rely on them exclusively. As an example, I once observed a primary care physician complete a case history on an elderly man. The doctor only asked questions that could be answered yes and no. The doctor asked, "Do you have high blood pressure, do you have diabetes, do you have thyroid problems? . . ." In each case the patient replied, "no." After firing a barrage of questions, the doctor prematurely concluded that the patient was in good health and proceeded with the physical exam. Later in the exam, the patient mentioned he had previously diagnosed liver cancer. The doctor was flustered because he had not elicited this crucial information earlier. He completely missed important information by asking specific yes-and-no questions. A more general question, such as, "Do you have any medical conditions?" would have likely revealed the cancer diagnosis. The point here is that a good case history in any language involves a mixture of open-ended and specific questions.

REGIONAL VARIATION OF SPANISH

Readers should keep in mind that not all Spanish-speaking countries use the same vocabulary for particular words and expressions.
For example, Spanish-speakers from the Americas call glasses *anteojos*
or *lentes*; Cubans and Puerto Ricans use the term *espejuelos*; and
people in Spain call them *gafas*. When possible, I have tried using
words and expressions understood by the vast majority of Spanish-
speakers. However, users will no doubt still encounter Spanish words
unique to their geographic location. For example, the preferred word
for "chin" may be *barba*, *barbilla*, or *menton*, depending on location.
Since it is not possible to detail every conceivable vocabulary preference, your best approach is to learn these details from your local
Spanish speakers.

VOLUNTEERS NEEDED

Several charitable organizations need eyecare professionals to
volunteer their services in Spanish-speaking countries. All provide
excellent exposure to Spanish-speaking patients while also offering
you the fulfillment of helping the underprivileged. These organizations
include Los Medicos Voladores (http://www.flyingdocs.org), Hospital de la
Familia (http://www.hospitaldelafamilia.org), and Volunteer Optometric
Services to Humanity International (http://www.vosh.org).

Acknowledgments

Oddly enough, *Spanish Terminology for the Eyecare Team* almost didn't happen. In 1999, a representative from the publisher, Butterworth-Heinemann (BH), was skeptical that my book would even sell. Yet through the persistence of Karen Oberheim, an editor at BH, they agreed to publish *Practical Spanish in Eyecare*. As a pleasant surprise, *Practical Spanish in Eyecare* sold well. In fact, it sold well enough that after Elsevier acquired BH, the title spawned similar books for dentistry, chiropractic, and other healthcare areas.

I thank Christie Hart, Senior Developmental Editor at Elsevier, for her leadership in the development of *Spanish Terminology for the Eyecare Team,* along with the other editors at Elsevier involved in this project. In light of the challenges getting the original book published, it is rewarding to see the fruition of my efforts.

I am very grateful to the many people involved in preparing the first edition; without their efforts, this second edition would not exist. Vernon Hammond, OD, contributed an extraordinary amount of time, drawing on his clinical expertise caring for a predominantly Spanish-speaking patient base. Words are inadequate to describe how much I admire Dr. Hammond's contribution to this work, as well as his dedication to the Spanish-speaking community. I also extend my appreciation to the members of the Salinas Valley Optometry Group and Hospital de la Familia. In particular, I thank Joseph Estrada, OD; Roberto Flores; Rosie Camp; Joan Ploem Miller, OD; S. Koontz, OD; Antonio Moran, OD; and Rosamaria Silva-Garcia. I thank Karen Oberheim, Cheri Dellelo, Jodie Allen, and the other editors at Butterworth-Heinemann involved in the original publication.

Finally, I acknowledge my wife, Kathryn. She has put up with the many evenings I have spent on this project.

Brian Chou, OD, FAAO
San Diego, California

How to Use this Book

Hispanic is a term used to identify people who speak the Spanish language and have Cuban, Central or South American, Mexican, or Puerto Rican backgrounds. The largest Hispanic populations in the United States reside in Arizona, California, Colorado, Florida, New Mexico, New York, and Texas. Since it is not possible to detail every conceivable vocabulary preference, this book uses a universally accepted dialect. However, you will probably still encounter some Spanish words unique to your area.

ORGANIZATION

The organization of this book follows a logical sequence of how a practitioner would interact with a patient. It starts with initial greeting and procedes through general and then to specialty appointments.

The book addresses the use of the formal "you" (usted) in situations among adults, and the appropriate use of the informal "you" (tú) in situations in which adults are addressing children.

In cases in which two or more words or phrases are appropriate, they are presented in parentheses and separated by a slash (/). In the following example, either the word "translator" or the word "interpreter" can be used to complete the sentence:

I need a (translator/interpreter)—wait a minute.

Necesito un (traductor/intérprete)—espere un minuto.

RESOURCES

We have included several resources that you may find helpful as you learn to communicate in Spanish.

A mini CD-ROM provides the English-to-Spanish translation of every phrase in the book. English phrases are spoken by an American elocutionist, and a Columbian elocutionist provides the Spanish phrases. Every phrase in the book is included. If your computer is set to Autorun, just load the CD-ROM into the drive. The CD-ROM will do the rest. The CD-ROM is compatible with both PC and Mac computers, but note that a tray-loading CD-ROM drive is required.

As part of this Resources section, we have included helpful information about the use of accents, verbs, nouns, and adjectives within the Spanish language. A pronunciation guide is also included. At the back of the book, an extensive English-to-Spanish glossary is provided for quick reference. The glossary is divided into categories such as eyecare terms, numbers, months of the year, etc. An alphabetical Spanish-to-English listing of each of the vocabulary words and a list of informal expressions used in conversation is also provided.

Accents*

Accentos

The acute accent is the only mark of its kind in Spanish. It is a small oblique line (á) that is drawn from right to left and specifies a syllable that has a stronger sound when pronouncing it. Accents are used generally to distinguish words written alike and identical in form with other parts of speech, but with a different meaning. For example: **papá** (father), **papa** (vegetable); **monté** (mounted), **monte** (large hill). Accents are sometimes omitted from capital letters.

El acento es la mayor intensidad con que se marca determinada sílaba al pronunciar una palabra. Es una rayita oblicua (á) que se escribe de derecha a izquierda y se coloca en ciertos casos sobre la vocal de la sílaba en que se carga la pronunciación. En español es muy necesario acentuar las palabras para darles el significado correcto que llevan. Por ejemplo: papá (**padre**), papa (**vegetal**); monté (**verbo**), monte (terreno elevado).

I love	amo
	(ah-moh)
he loved	él amó
	(ehl ah-moh)
the owner	el dueño/amo
	(ehl doo-eh-nyoh/ah-moh)
road	el camino
	(ehl kah-mee-noh)
he walked	él caminó
	(ehl kah-mee-noh)
copper	cobre
	(koh-breh)
I charged	yo cobré
	(yoh koh-breh)
volumes	volúmenes
	(boh-loo-meh-nehs)

---

* From Joyce EV, Villanueva ME: Say it in Spanish, ed 2. Philadelphia, Saunders, 2000.

never	jamás
	(hah-mahs)
pencil	lápiz
	(lah-pees)

Nouns

Sustantivos

GENDER OF NOUNS*
GÈNERO DE LOS SUSTANTIVOS

In Spanish, the gender of a noun corresponds to sex. The name of any male being is masculine; that of a female being is feminine. The grammatical gender of an inanimate object must simply be memorized: a bone (el hueso) is masculine, the head (la cabeza) is feminine, and so on.

En español, el género de los sustantivos corresponde al sexo. El nombre de un hombre es masculino, el de una mujer es femenino. El género gramatical de un objeto inanimado se debe memorizar: un hueso es masculino, la cabeza es femenina y asÍ sucesivamente.

All Spanish nouns must be masculine or feminine.

The definite article *the* has the following singular and plural forms in Spanish.

el (singular masculine)   la (singular feminine)
los (plural masculine)   las (plural feminine)

The indefinite article *a* or *an* has the following forms in Spanish.

un (singular masculine)   una (singular feminine)
unos (plural masculine)   unas (plural feminine)

Masculine nouns require a masculine article; feminine nouns require a feminine article.

the man	el hombre
	(ehl ohm-breh)
the woman	la mujer
	(lah moo-hehr)
the boy	el muchacho
	(ehl moo-chah-choh)
the back	la espalda
	(lah ehs-pahl-dah)
the friend	el amigo
	(ehl ah-mee-goh)

---

* From Joyce EV, Villanueva ME: Say it in Spanish, ed 2. Philadelphia, Saunders, 2000.

xix

a rib	una costilla
	(oo-nah kohs-tee-yah)
the eye	el ojo
	(ehl oh-hoh)
a skeleton	un esqueleto
	(oon ehs-keh-leh-toh)
the clavicle	la clavÍcula
	(lah klah-bee-koo-lah)

Nouns ending in -al, -ante, -ador, -ón, and -o are usually masculine.

An important exception is **la mano**. In spite of the ending *o*, *la mano* is feminine.

the hospital	el hospital
	(ehl ohs-pee-tahl)
the tranquilizer	el tranquilizante
	(ehl trahn-kee-lee-sahn-teh)
the worker	el trabajador
	(ehl trah-bah-hah-dohr)
the heart	el corazón
	(ehl koh-rah-sohn)

The days of the week, months of the year, and the names of languages are masculine.

Wednesday	el miércoles
	(ehl mee-ehr-koh-lehs)
the month of April	el mes de abril
	(ehl mehs deh ah-breel)
Spanish	el español
	(ehl ehs-pah-nyohl)

Nouns ending in -tad, -dad, -ción, -sión, -ez, -ie, -ud, and -umbre are usually feminine.

the dehydration	la deshidratación
	(lah deh-see-drah-tah-see-ohn)
the habit	la costumbre
	(lah kohs-toom-breh)
the age	la edad
	(lah eh-dahd)
the friendship	la amistad
	(lah ah-mees-tahd)
the series	la serie
	(lah seh-ree-eh)
the health	la salud
	(lah sah-lood)

Nouns ending in -e should be memorized with the definite article.

the blood   la sangre
                                           (lah sahn-greh)

PLURAL OF NOUNS

A noun ending in a vowel forms the plural by adding **-s**; those ending in a consonant add **-es**.

the physician   el médico
                                           (ehl meh-dee-koh)
the physicians   los médicos
                                           (lohs meh-dee-kohs)
the doctor   el doctor
                                           (ehl dohk-tohr)
the doctors   los doctores
                                           (lohs dohk-toh-rehs)

A noun ending in **-z** changes to **-c** and then adds **-es**.

the nose   la nariz
                                           (lah nahr-ees)
the noses   las narices
                                           (lahs nahr-ee-sehs)

Nouns ending in a stressed vowel form the plural by adding **-es**.

the ruby   el rubí
                                           (ehl roo-bee)
the rubies   los rubíes
                                           (lohs roo-bee-ehs)

Nouns ending in unstressed **-es** or **-is** are considered to be both singular and plural. Number is expressed by the article.

Thursday   el jueves
                                           (ehl hoo-eh-behs)
Thursdays   los jueves
                                           (lohs hoo-eh-behs)

SPECIAL USES OF ARTICLES

The definite article is used in Spanish but omitted in English as follows:

1. Before the names of languages, except after **hablar**, **en**, or **de**:

Spanish is important.   El español es importante.
                                           (ehl ehs-pah-nyohl ehs eem-
                                               pohr-tahn-teh)

My friend speaks French.

Mi amigo habla francés.
(mee ah-mee-goh ah-blah
frahn-sehs)

The whole book is
in German.

Todo el libro está en alemán.
(toh-doh ehl lee-broh ehs-
tah ehn ah-eh-mahn)

2. Before titles, except when addressing the person:

Mr. Gomez left yesterday.

El señor Gómez salió ayer.
(ehl seh-nyohr goh-mehs
sah-lee-oh ah-yehr)

How are you, Mrs. García?

Cómo está, señora García?
(koh-moh ehs-tah, seh-nyoh-
rah gahr-see-ah)

The article is omitted before **don**, **doña**, **Santo**, **Santa**, **San**.

3. With parts of the body or personal possessions (e.g., clothing):

He has black hair.

El tiene pelo negro.
(ehl tee-eh-neh peh-loh
neh-groh)

Mary has a broken foot.

María tiene el pie quebrado.
(mah-ree-ah tee-eh-neh ehl
pee-eh keh-brah-doh)

4. With the time of day (la hora, the hour; las horas, the hours):

It is one o'clock.

Es la una.
(ehs lah oo-nah)

I go to sleep at eleven.

Me duermo a las once.
(meh doo-ehr-moh ah lahs
ohn-seh)

5. With the names of seasons:

I like summer.

Me gusta el verano.
(meh goos-tah ehl beh-
rah-noh)

6. With the days of the week, except after the verb ser (to be):

I go downtown
(on) Tuesdays.

Los martes voy al centro.
(lohs mahr-tehs boy ahl
sehn-troh)

Today is Monday.

Hoy es lunes.
(oh-ee ehs loo-nehs)

7. Before certain geographic areas:

Canada

el Canadá
(ehl kah-nah-dah)

Argentina

la Argentina
(lah ahr-hehn-tee-nah)

NEUTER ARTICLE *LO*

1. The neuter article **lo** precedes an adjective used as a noun to express a quality or an abstract idea.

I like red (that which is red).
Me gusta lo rojo.
(meh goos-tah loh roh-hoh)

I think the same as you.
Pienso lo mismo que usted.
(pee-ehn-soh loh mees-moh keh oos-tehd)

2. **Lo** + adjective or adverb + **que** = *how.*

I see how good she is.
Ya veo lo buena que es.
(yah beh-oh loh boo-eh-nah keh ehs)

Since the article **lo** is neuter, it has no plural form. Therefore, **lo** is used whether the adjective is masculine or feminine, singular or plural.

OMISSION OF ARTICLES

1. The definite article is omitted in the following cases.
   A. Before nouns in a position:
      Austin, the capital of Texas, is at the center of the state.
      Austin, capital de Texas, está en el centro del estado.
   B. Before numerals expressing the numerical order of rulers:

Charles the Fifth
Carlos Quinto
(kahr-lohs keen-toh)

Mary the Second
María Segunda
(mah-ree-ah seh-goon-dah)

2. The indefinite article is omitted before predicate nouns denoting a class or group (social class, occupation, nationality, religion, etc.):

He is a barber.
Es barbero.
(ehs bahr-beh-roh)

I am Mexican.
Soy mexicana.
(soh-ee meh-hee-kah-nah)

I want to be a nurse.
Quiero ser enfermera.
(kee-eh-roh sehr ehn-fehr-meh-rah)

If the predicate noun is modified, the indefinite article is stated:

He is a hard-working barber.
Es un barbero muy trabajador.
(ehs oon bahr-beh-roh moo-ee trah-bah-hah-dohr)

I want to be a good nurse.

Quiero ser una buena
enfermera.
(kee-eh-roh sehr oo-nah
boo-eh-nah ehn-fehr-
meh-rah)

Adjectives and Pronouns*

Adjetivos y Pronombres

Adjectives describe nouns and pronouns. In Spanish, adjectives are placed after the noun. They agree in number and gender with the noun they modify.

ADJECTIVES ENDING IN -o/-a

Masculine singular:

The patient is happy.
El paciente está contento.
(ehl pah-see-ehn-teh ehs-tah
  kohn-tehn-toh)

Feminine singular:

She is happy.
Ella está contenta.
(eh-yah ehs-tah kohn-
  tehn-tah)

Masculine plural:

They are happy.
Ellos están contentos.
(eh-yohs ehs-tahn kohn-
  tehn-tohs)

Feminine plural:

They are happy.
Ellas están contentas.
(eh-yahs ehs-tahn kohn-
  tehn-tahs)

ADJECTIVES ENDING IN -e

Masculine singular:

He is sad.
El está triste.
(ehl ehs-tah trees-teh)

Feminine singular:

She is sad.
Ella está triste.
(eh-yah ehs-tah trees-teh)

---

* From Joyce EV, Villanueva ME: Say it in Spanish, ed 2. Philadelphia, Saunders, 2000.

Masculine plural:
They are sad.
Ellos están tristes.
(eh-yohs ehs-tahn trees-tehs)

Feminine plural:
They are sad.
Ellas están tristes.
(eh-yahs ehs-tahn trees-tehs)

ADJECTIVES ENDING IN A CONSONANT

Masculine singular:
The procedure is difficult.
El procedimiento es difícil.
(ehl proh-seh-dee-mee-ehn-
toh ehs dee-fee-seel)

Feminine singular:
The measurement is difficult.
La medida es difícil.
(lah meh-dee-dah ehs dee-
fee-seel)

Masculine plural:
The exams are difficult.
Los exámenes son difíciles.
(lohs ehx-ah-meh-nehs sohn
dee-fee-see-lehs)

Feminine plural:
The measurements are
difficult.
Las medidas son difíciles.
(lahs meh-dee-dahs sohn
dee-fee-see-lehs)

Demonstrative adjectives precede the nouns they modify and agree with them in number and gender.

this book
este libro
(ehs-teh lee-broh)

these pens
estas plumas
(ehs-tahs ploo-mahs)

Este (*this*) refers to what is near or directly concerns me.

Esos (*those*) refers to what is near or directly concerns you.

Aquel (*that*) refers to what is remote to the speaker or the person addressed.

This pencil is red.
Este lápiz es rojo.
(ehs-teh lah-pees ehs
roh-hoh)

John, give me that bone.
Juan, déme aquel hueso.
(hoo-ahn, deh-meh ah-kehl
oo-eh-soh)

SOME COMMON LIMITING ADJECTIVES

all, everything	todo (toh-doh)
bad	malo (mah-loh)
better	mejor (meh-hohr)
big (age)	grande (grahn-deh)
first	primero (pree-meh-roh)
fourth	cuarto (koo-ahr-toh)
good	bueno (boo-eh-noh)
less	menos (meh-nohs)
little, few	poco (poh-koh)
more	mucho, más (moo-choh, mahs)
nothing	nada (nah-dah)
one, a, an	un (oon)
small (age, fit)	pequeño/chico (peh-keh-nyoh/chee-koh)

POSSESSIVE PRONOUNS

	Singular	Plural
mine	el mío, la mía (ehl mee-oh, lah mee-ah)	los míos, las mías (lohs mee-ohs, lahs mee-ahs)
yours	el tuyo, la tuya (ehl too-yoh, lah too-yah)	los tuyos, las tuyas (lohs too-yohs, lahs too-yahs)
his, hers, theirs	el suyo, la suya (ehl soo-yoh, lah soo-yah)	los suyos, las suyas (lohs soo-yohs, lahs soo-yahs)
ours	el nuestro, la nuestra (ehl noo-ehs-troh, lah noo-ehs-trah)	los nuestros, las nuestras (lohs noo-ehs-trohs, lahs noo-ehs-trahs)

Possessive pronouns are formed by the definite article plus the long form of the possessive adjective.

My nose is prettier than yours.	Mi nariz es más bonita que la tuya.
	(mee nah-rees ehs mahs boh-nee-tah keh lah too-yah)

After the verb **ser**, the article preceding the possessive pronoun is generally omitted.

The bones are mine.	Los huesos son míos.
	(lohs oo-eh-sohs soh mee-ohs)
That gown is yours.	Aquella bata es suya.
	(ah-keh-yah bah-tah ehs soo-yah)
These books are mine.	Estos libros son míos.
	(ehs-tohs lee-brohs sohn mee-ohs)

Possession is expressed by **de** + the possessor. This corresponds to 's or s' in English.

his pens and yours	sus plumas y las de usted
	(soos ploo-mahs ee lahs deh oos-tehd)
Martin's pencil	el lápiz de Martín
	(ehl lah-pees deh mahr-teen)
my book and Louisa's	mi libro y el de Luisa
	(mee lee-broh ee ehl deh loo-ee-sah)
our patient	nuestro paciente
	(noo-ehs-troh pah-see-ehn-teh)
her rings	sus anillos
	(soos ah-nee-yohs)
a friend of theirs	un amigo de ellos
	(oon ah-mee-goh deh eh-yohs)

WHOSE?

The interrogative pronoun *whose?* is expressed in Spanish by **de quién es?**

Whose pen is it?	¿De quién es la pluma?
	(deh kee-ehn ehs lah ploo-mah)

It belongs to the doctor.	Es del doctor.
	(ehs dehl dohk-tohr)
Whose card is it?	¿De quién es la tarjeta?
	(deh kee-ehn ehs lah tahr-heh-tah)
Mr. García's.	Del señor García.
	(dehl seh-nyohr gahr-see-ah)
Whose x-rays are these?	¿De quién son estas radiografías?
	(deh kee-ehn sohn ehs-tahs rah-dee-oh-grah-fee-ahs)
They are Mrs. Luna's.	Son de la señora Luna.
	(sohn deh lah seh-nyoh-rah loo-nah)

SOME COMMON PREPOSITIONS

about	acerca de
	(ah-sehr-kah deh)
according	según
	(seh-goon)
after	después de
	(dehs-poo-ehs deh)
against	contra
	(kohn-trah)
among, between	entre
	(ehn-treh)
around	alrededor de
	(ahl-reh-deh-dohr deh)
before	antes de
	(ahn-tehs deh)
behind	detrás de
	(deh-trahs deh)
beneath, under	debajo de
	(deh-bah-hoh deh)
beside	además de
	(ah-deh-mahs deh)
during	durante
	(doo-rahn-teh)
far	lejos de
	(leh-hohs deh)

for	para
	(pah-rah)
for, by, therefore	por
	(pohr)
from, of	de
	(deh)
in	en
	(ehn)
in front of	enfrente de
	(ehn-frehn-teh deh)
in front of	delante de
	(deh-lahn-teh deh)
near	cerca de
	(sehr-kah deh)
outside of	fuera de
	(foo-eh-rah deh)
over, above	sobre
	(soh-breh)
since	desde
	(dehs-deh)
to, at	a
	(ah)
toward	hacia
	(ah-see-ah)
until	hasta
	(ahs-tah)
with	con
	(kohn)
within	dentro de
	(dehn-troh deh)

TABLE 1 Feminine and Masculine Adjectives	TABLA 1 Adjetivos femeninos y masculinos
English	**Spanish**
Feminine	*Masculine*
this esta (ehs-tah)	este (ehs-teh)
these estas (ehs-tahs)	estos (ehs-tohs)
that esa (eh-sah)	ese (eh-seh)
those esas (eh-sahs)	esos (eh-sohs)
that aquella (ah-keh-yah)	aquel (ah-kehl)
those aquellas (ah-keh-yahs)	aquellos (ah-keh-yohs)

TABLE 2 Personal Pronouns		TABLA 2 Pronombres personales	
Singular		**Plural**	
English	*Spanish*	*English*	*Spanish*
I	yo (yoh)	we (masculine)	nosotros (noh-soh-trohs)
		we (feminine)	nosotras (noh-soh-trahs)
you (familiar)	tú (too)	you	vosotros/as (boh-soh-trohs/ahs)
you (formal)	usted (oos-tehd)	you	ustedes (oos-teh-dehs)
he	él (ehl)	they (masculine)	ellos (eh-yohs)
she	ella (eh-yah)	they (feminine)	ellas (eh-yahs)

Verbs

Verbos

Verbs are to a sentence what the spinal cord is to the body. Verbs give structure to a sentence because they tell us what is being done and when it is being done; for example: I *talk* to the nurse (present), I *talked* to the nurse (past), I *will talk* to the nurse (future).

Los verbos son para una oración lo que la espina dorsal es para el cuerpo. Los verbos dan estructura a una oración al indicar qué es lo que se está haciendo y cuándo se está haciendo; por ejemplo: Yo *hablo* con la enfermera (presente), Yo *hablé* con la enfermera ayer (pasado), Yo *hablaré* con la enfermera mañana (futuro).

Regular verbs end in **-ar**, **-er**, or **-ir** in Spanish. They are easy to conjugate because you usually take the stem of the verb and add the endings: **o, as, a, amos, an**. See Table 1.

Los verbos regulares tienen la terminación -ar, -er, o -ir en español. Son fáciles de conjugarse ya que usualmente se toma la raíz del verbo y se le agrega la terminación: o, as, a, amos, -an. Vea la Tabla 1.

to auscultate	auscultar (ah-oos-kool-tahr)
to be born	nacer (nah-sehr)
to become ill	enfermarse (ehn-fehr-mahr-seh)
to bring near	acercar (ah-sehr-kahr)
to call	llamar (yah-mahr)
to die	morir (moh-reer)
to eat	comer (koh-mehr)
to examine	examinar (ehx-ah-mee-nahr)

to get better	mejorar
	(meh-hoh-rahr)
to heal	sanar
	(sah-nahr)
to hear	oír
	(oh-eer)
to hurt	doler
	(doh-lehr)
to leave (behind)	dejar
	(deh-hahr)
to listen	escuchar
	(ehs-koo-chahr)
to live	vivir
	(bee-beer)
to name	nombrar
	(nohm-brahr)
to operate	operar
	(oh-peh-rahr)
to palpate	palpar
	(pahl-pahr)
to revise	revisar
	(reh-bee-sahr)
to see	ver
	(behr)
to vomit	vomitar
	(boh-mee-tahr)
to agree	acordar
	(ah-kohr-dahr)
to bore	aburrir
	(ah-boo-reer)
to come	venir
	(beh-neer)
to deserve	merecer
	(meh-reh-sehr)
to finish	acabar
	(ah-kah-bahr)
to go out	salir
	(sah-leer)
to let go	soltar
	(sohl-tahr)
to need	necesitar
	(neh-seh-see-tahr)

to reach	alcanzar
	(ahl-kahn-sahr)
to remain	quedar
	(keh-dahr)
to stop	parar
	(pah-rahr)
to take out	sacar
	(sah-kahr)
to walk	caminar
	(kah-mee-nahr)

Personal pronouns designate who is performing the action. Many times it is not necessary to include the personal pronouns when conjugating a verb or using it in a sentence.

Los pronombres personales designan a las personas que hacen la acción. Muchas veces no es necesario usar la persona al conjugar verbos o al usarlos en una oración.

PERSONAL PRONOUNS

I	yo
	(yoh)
you (*informal*)	tú
	(too)
he/she/you (*formal*)	él/ella/usted
	(ehl/eh-yah/oos-tehd)
we	nosotros
	(noh-soh-trohs)
you (*plural*)	ustedes
they	ellos/ellas
	(eh-yohs/eh-yahs/oos-teh-dehs)

To Feel	**Sentir**
	(Sehn-Teer)
I feel	siento
	(see-ehn-toh)
you (*informal*) feel	sientes
	(see-ehn-tehs)
he/she feels; you (*formal*) feel	siente
	(see-ehn-teh)
we feel	sentimos
	(sehn-tee-mohs)

they feel	sienten
	(see-ehn-tehn)

To Sit Down — **Sentarse (Sehn-Tahr-Seh)**

I sit	me siento
	(meh see-ehn-toh)
you (*informal*) sit	te sientas
	(teh see-ehn-tahs)
he/she sits; you (*formal*) sit	se sienta
	(seh see-ehn-tah)
we sit	nos sentamos
	(nohs sehn-tah-mohs)
they sit	se sientan
	(seh see-ehn-tahn)

The reflexive pronouns change the verb's action.

Los pronombres reflexivos cambian la acción del verbo.

Mover (To Move)

Action On Self	**Action On Object**
yo me muevo	yo muevo
(yoh meh moo-eh-boh)	(yoh moo-eh-boh)
tú te mueves	tú mueves
(too teh moo-eh-behs)	(too moo-eh-behs)
él/ella se mueve	él/ella mueve
(ehl/eh-yah seh moo-eh-beh)	(ehl/eh-yah moo-eh-beh)
nosotros nos movemos	nosotros movemos
(noh-soh-trohs nohs moh-beh-mohs)	(noh-soh-trohs moh-beh-mohs)
ellos/ellas se mueven	ellos/ellas mueven
(eh-yohs/eh-yahs seh moo-eh-behn)	(eh-yohs/eh-yahs moo-eh-behn)
to advise	aconsejar
	(ah-kohn-seh-hahr)
to ask	preguntar
	(preh-goon-tahr)
to bathe	bañar
	(bah-nyahr)
to be afraid	temer
	(teh-mehr)
to believe	creer
	(kreh-ehr)

to boil	hervir (ehr-beer)
to break	romper (rohm-pehr)
to build	construir (kohns-troo-eer)
to carry	llevar (yeh-bahr)
to change	cambiar (kahm-bee-ahr)
to clean	limpiar (leem-pee-ahr)
to communicate	comunicar (koh-moo-nee-kahr)
to complain	quejar (keh-hahr)
to conduct	conducir (kohn-doo-seer)
to confuse	confundir (kohn-foon-deer)
to cook	cocinar (koh-see-nahr)
to cover	cubrir (koo-breer)
to cry	llorar (yoh-rahr)
to cut	cortar (kohr-tahr)
to deny	negar (neh-gahr)
to destroy	destruir (dehs-troo-eer)
to disappear	desaparecer (deh-sah-pah-reh-sehr)
to discover, find	descubrir (dehs-koo-breer)
to do/make	hacer (ah-sehr)
to drink	beber (beh-behr)
to eat breakfast	desayunar (deh-sah-yoo-nahr)

to embrace	abrazar
	(ah-brah-sahr)
to employ	emplear
	(ehm-pleh-ahr)
to feel	sentir
	(sehn-teer)
to fill	llenar
	(yeh-nahr)
to find	hallar
	(ah-yahr)
to fix	componer
	(kohm-poh-nehr)
to fly	volar
	(boh-lahr)
to get up, raise	levantar
	(leh-bahn-tahr)
to give	dar
	(dahr)
to go	ir
	(eer)
to go to bed, lie down	acostarse
	(ah-kohs-tahr-seh)
to have	haber
	(ah-behr)
to hunt	cazar
	(kah-sahr)
to joke, kid	bromear
	(broh-meh-ahr)
to jump	saltar
	(sahl-tahr)
to kiss	besar
	(beh-sahr)
to know	conocer
	(koh-noh-sehr)
to lose	perder
	(pehr-dehr)
to marry	casar
	(kah-sahr)
to paint	pintar
	(peen-tahr)
to point	señalar
	(seh-nyah-lahr)

to promise	prometer (proh-meh-tehr)
to receive	recibir (reh-see-beer)
to recognize	reconocer (reh-koh-noh-sehr)
to remember	acordar/recordar (ah-kohr-dahr/reh-kohr-dahr)
to respond	responder (rehs-pohn-dehr)
to return	regresar/volver (reh-greh-sahr/bohl-behr)
to scream	gritar (gree-tahr)
to see	ver (behr)
to sell	vender (behn-dehr)
to serve	servir (sehr-beer)
to shake	temblar (tehm-blahr)
to sit	sentar (sehn-tahr)
to sleep	dormir (dohr-meer)
to speak	hablar (ah-blahr)
to start	comenzar (koh-mehn-sahr)
to step	pisar (pee-sahr)
to suffer	sufrir (soo-freer)
to take	tomar (toh-mahr)
to thank for	agradecer (ah-grah-deh-sehr)
to try	tratar (trah-tahr)
to turn	voltear (bohl-teh-ahr)

to turn off	apagar
	(ah-pah-gahr)
to want	querer
	(keh-rehr)
to wash	lavar
	(lah-bahr)
to wish	desear
	(deh-seh-ahr)
to work	trabajar
	(trah-bah-hahr)
to accept	aceptar
	(ah-sehp-tahr)
to activate	activar
	(ahk-tee-bahr)
to administer	administrar
	(ahd-mee-nees-trahr)
to authorize	autorizar
	(ah-oo-toh-ree-sahr)
to beat, knock	golpear
	(gohl-peh-ahr)
to bleed	sangrar
	(sahn-grahr)
to conserve	conservar
	(kohn-sehr-bahr)
to control	controlar
	(kohn-troh-lahr)
to evaluate	evaluar
	(eh-bah-loo-ahr)
to hit	pegar
	(peh-gahr)
to inform	informar
	(een-fohr-mahr)
to interpret	interpretar
	(een-tehr-preh-tahr)
to present	presentar
	(preh-sehn-tahr)
to protect	protejer
	(proh-teh-hehr)
to provoke	provocar
	(proh-boh-kahr)
to reduce	reducir
	(reh-doo-seer)

to revise	revisar
	(reh-bee-sahr)
to select	seleccionar
	(seh-lehk-see-oh-nahr)
to separate	separar
	(seh-pah-rahr)
to suspend	suspender
	(soos-pehn-dehr)
to write	escribir
	(ehs-kree-beer)

TO *BE* VERBS

The verbs **ser** and **estar** both translate in English as *to be*, but they are not interchangeable. Both are irregular in the present and the past tense.

Los verbos *ser* y *estar* se traducen al inglés *to be*, pero no se intercambian. Los dos verbos son irregulares en el tiempo presente y en el pasado.

	Ser	**Estar**
I am	yo soy	yo estoy
	(yo soh-ee)	(yoh ehs-tohy)
you (*informal*) are	usted es/tú eres	usted está/tú estás
	(oos-tehd ehs-too eh-rehs)	(oos-tehd ehs-tah/ too ehs-tahs)
he/she/it is	él/ella/eso es	él/ella/eso está
	(ehl/eh-yah/eh- soh ehs)	(ehl/eh-yah/eh-soh ehs-tah)
we are	nosotros somos	nosotros estamos
	(noh-soh-trohs soh-mohs)	(noh-soh-trohs ehs-tah-mohs)
they are	ellos/ellas son	ellos/ellas están
	(eh-yohs/eh-yahs sohn)	(eh-yohs/eh-yahs ehs-tahn)

USES OF *SER*

Ser expresses a relatively permanent quality.

age:	You are old.	Usted es viejo.
characteristic:	The snow is cold.	La nieve es fría.
color:	The urine is yellow.	La orina es amarilla.

shape:	The glass is round.	El vaso es redondo.
size:	You are tall.	Usted es alto.
possession:	The pencil is mine.	El lápiz es mío.
wealth:	The man is rich.	El hombre es rico.

Ser is used with predicate nouns, pronouns, or adjectives.

He is a dentist.	El es dentista
Who am I?	¿Quién soy yo?
We are Protestant.	Nosotros somos protestantes.

Ser indicates material, origin, or ownership.

material:	The needle is metal.	La aguja es de metal.
origin:	The doctor is from Texas.	El doctor es de Tejas.
ownership:	The dentures are mine.	Las dentaduras son mías.

Ser tells time.

It is one o'clock.	Es la una.
It is 10 o'clock.	Son las diez.

USES OF *ESTAR*

Estar expresses location (permanent and temporary).

Dallas is in Texas.	Dallas está en Tejas.
I am in the room.	Yo estoy en el cuarto.

Estar expresses status of health.

How are you?	¿Cómo está usted?
I am fine.	Estoy bien.
We are sick.	Estamos enfermos.

Estar expresses a temporary characteristic or quality.

He is nervous.	El está nervioso.
I am ready.	Estoy lista.
You are far away.	Usted está lejos.

TABLE 3 Regular Verb		TABLA 3 Verbo regular	
Verb	**Stem**	**Ending**	**Persons**
To live	viv-	o	yo vivo (yoh bee-boh)
Vivir (bee-beer)	viv-	es	tú vives (too bee-behs)
	viv-	e	el/ella vive (ehl/eh-yah bee-beh)
	viv-	imos	nosotros vivimos (noh-soh-trohs bee-bee-mohs)
	viv-	en	ellos/ellas viven (eh-yohs/eh-yahs bee-behn)

TABLE 4 **Present and Past Tense**	**TABLA 4** **Tiempo presente y pasado**

VERB: to eat	**comer (koh-mehr)**
Present Tense	*Tiempo presente*
I eat	yo como (yoh koh-moh)
you eat	tú comes (too koh-mehs)
he/she eats	él/ella come (ehl/eh-yah koh-meh)
we eat	nosotros comemos (noh-soh- trohs koh-meh-mohs)
they eat	ellos/ellas comen (eh-yohs/ eh-yahs koh-mehn)
Past Tense	*Tiempo pasado*
I ate	yo comí (yoh koh-mee)
you ate	tú comiste (too koh-mees-teh)
he/she ate	él/ella comió (ehl/eh-yah koh-mee-oh)
we ate	nosotros comimos (noh-soh- trohs koh-mee-mohs)
they ate	ellos/ellas comi l eron (eh-yohs/ eh-yahs koh-mee-eh-rohn)

TABLE 5
Verb Tenses

TABLA 5
Tiempo de los verbos

Verb: To speak

Present Tense	*Tiempo presente*
to speak	hablar (ah-blahr)
I speak	yo hablo (yoh ah-bloh)
you speak	tú hablas (too ah-blahs)
he/she speaks	él/ella habla (ehl/eh-yah ah-blah)
we speak	nosotros hablamos (noh-soh-trohs ah-blah-mohs)
they speak	ellos/ellas hablan (eh-yohs/eh-yahs ah-blahn)

Past Tense	*Tiempo pasado*
I spoke	yo hablé (yoh ah-bleh)
you spoke	tú hablaste (too ah-blahs-teh)
he/she spoke	él/ella habló (ehl/eh-yah ah-bloh)
we spoke	nosotros hablamos (noh-soh-trohs ah-blah-mohs)
they spoke	ellos/ellas hablaron (eh-yohs/eh-yahs ah-blah-rohn)

Future Tense	*Tiempo futuro*
I will speak	yo hablaré (yoh ah-blah-reh)
you will speak	tú hablarás (too ah-blah-rahs)
he/she will speak	él/ella hablará (ehl/eh-yah ah-blah-rah)
we will speak	nosotros hablaremos (noh-soh-trohs ah-blah-reh-mohs)
they will speak	ellos/ellas hablarán (eh-yohs/eh-yahs ah-blah-rahn)

A sounds like *a* in *father* and is pronounced like a clipped *ah*.

ayudar	to help
el abdomen	abdomen
la amígdala	tonsil
la cama	bed
la bata	bathrobe

B has the sound of *b* in book when it begins a sentence and when it follows *m* or *n*.

el bol	basin
bañar	to bathe
el brazo	arm
el hombre	man
la boca	mouth

The sound of **B** becomes softened when it is located between vowels.

la cabeza	head
el rebozo	shawl

The Spanish **B** and **V** have the same sound.

C has a hard sound, as in *come* when it occurs before *a, o, u,* or before a consonant.

la cama	bed
la cuna	cradle
el cuello	neck
la cara	face

C before an *e* or *i* has an *s* sound.

la medicina	medicine
ciego	blind
la receta	prescription
la cintura	waist
el cerebro	brain

CH has the sound of *ch* in child.

el muchacho	boy
chupar	to suck
la noche	night

la chaqueta	jacket
la chica	girl
el chupón	pacifier

D has a hard sound as in *dental* at the beginning of a word.

la debilidad	weakness
los dientes	teeth
el doctor	doctor
mandar	to order
el dolor	pain

D has a soft or *th* sound as in *them* between vowels.

el lado	side
el médico	doctor
el dedo	finger
el cuidado	care
el codo	elbow
mojado	wet

E sounds like the English e in the word *eight*.

el pecho	chest
el pelo	hair
la enfermedad	illness
la espalda baja	lower back
eructar	to belch
el bébe	baby
la espalda	back
el papel	paper
el equilibrio	equilibrium
la mesa	table
estornudar	to sneeze
el estómago	stomach
empujar	to push

F has the same sounds as in English.

la fiebre	fever
frío	cold temperature
la fecha	date on the calendar
fumar	to smoke
flaco	skinny

G before *a, o,* or *u* has a hard sound in *get*.

Gordo	fat
las gafas	eyeglasses
el gargajo	phlegm
el gato	cat

G before an *e* or *i* has a guttural *h* sound as in the German *ach*.

la gente	people
las alergias	allergies
las gemelos	twins

Occasionally a silent *u* will precede the *e* or *i* to indicate that the **G** is hard, as in *go*.

pagué	paid
el hormigueo	tingling sensation or "pins and needles"

To keep the *u* sound in the *-gue* or *-gui* combination, a dieresis (¨) is placed over the *u*:

la vergüenza	shame
el ungüento	ointment

H is a silent letter.

humano	human
hinchar	to swell
las hormonas	hormones
el hueso	bone
el hígado	liver
el huevo	egg

I is a short sound as in *machine*.

irritable	irritable
la incisión	incision
el instrumento	instrument
incómodo	uncomfortable
mi	my

J sounds like a hard English *h*, a guttural *h* sound as in the German *ach*.

la jeringa	syringe
las orejas	ears
el jaunete	bunion
los ojos	eyes
la aguja	needle
trabajar	to work

K is not part of the Spanish alphabet. It is used only in words of foreign origin, and it has the same pronunciation as in English.

el kilo	kilogram
el kilómetro	kilometer

L is the same as in English.

la lengua	tongue
la píldora	pill

el líquido	liquid
las lágrimas	tears
los labios	lips
la luz	light

LL sounds like *y* in the word *yes*.

los tobillos	ankles
llorar	to cry
la cuchillada	gash
las costillas	ribs
la espaldilla	shoulder blade
la mejilla	cheek

M is the same as in English.

Morir	to die
las manos	hands
la médula	marrow
el músculo	muscle

N is pronounced like *m* before *b, f, p, m*, and *v*.

enfermo	sick
la enfermera	nurse
un brazo	arm
un viejo	old man
un pulmón	lung

N otherwise sounds the same as in English.

la náusea	nausea
nervioso	nervous
la nariz	nose
nacer	to be born

Ñ has the English sound of *ny* or *ni* as in *canyon* or *onion*.

los riñones	kidneys
el puño	fist
estreñido	constipated
el sueño	dream, sleep
el señor	Mr., the gentleman, sir
la muñeca	wrist

O sounds like the *o* in *born*.

la obesidad	obesity
la oreja	ear
emocional	emotional
el muslo	thigh
no	no
el pelo	hair

O followed by a consonant sounds like the English *o* in *or*.

orinar	to urinate
el ombligo	navel
el órgano	organ

P has the same sound as in English.

la parálisis	paralysis
el pañal	diaper
poco	little, referring to quantity
el paciente	patient
la pulmonía	pneumonia
el papá	dad
puje	bear down

Sometimes, **P** is silent, as in:

la psicología	psychology
la psiquiatra	psychiatrist
la psicoterapia	psychotherapy

Q appears only before *ue* or *ui*. The *u* is always silent, and the **Q** has a *k* sound.

Quejar	to complain
tranquilo	tranquil
la quijada	jaw
la izquierda	left
los bronquios	bronchial tubes
el queso	cheese

R is trilled at the beginning of a word.

la roncha	rash
el reumatismo	rheumatism
las rodillas	knees
el resfriado, el resfrío	cold in the nose

R is slightly trilled in the middle of a word.

primo	cousin
la varicela	chicken pox
la hernia	hernia
operar	to operate
la nariz	nose

RR is strongly trilled.

el carro	car
el catarro	cold in the head
el perro	dog

S has the *ess* sound of English.

la saliva	saliva
toser	to cough

el sarampión	measles
la causa	cause
el sudor	sweat
la sangre	blood
la vista	sight, vision

S before *b, d, g, l, m, n,* and *v* has a z sound, as in *toys.*

el asma	asthma
los dientes	teeth
la desgana	loss of appetite

T is similar to English.

el té	tea
tragar	to swallow
las tijeras	scissors
el teléfono	telephone
tranquilo	tranquil
este	this

U sounds like the English *u* in *rule.*

último	last in a series
usar	to use
la unión	union
único	only

V has the same sound as *b* in Spain. In most Latin countries *v* sounds like *v.*

el vértigo	dizziness
vestirse	to get dressed
la verruga	wart
el vientre	belly
aliviarse	to get well

W is not part of the Spanish alphabet. It is used only in foreign words and is pronounced as it is in English.

Wáshington	Washington

X has the sound of English *x* before a consonant.

explicar	to explain
la extensión	extension
excelente	excellent
el extranjero	foreigner

When it stands between vowels, **X** has a gs sound as in *eggs.*

el examen	exam
el oxÍgeno	oxygen

Y sounds like the English *y* in *yes.*

yo	I
el yodo	iodine

yeso	cast
el yerno	son-in-law

When **Y** follows *n*, it has the sound as the English *j* as in *judge*.

la inyección	injection
inyectar	to inject

When **Y** stands alone (meaning "and"), it sounds like the Spanish *i*.
Z always has the *s* sound.

el zumbido	buzzing
embarazada	pregnant
el corazón	heart
izquierdo	left
el brazo	arm
zurdo	left-handed
el zapato	shoe
la matriz	womb

GREETING THE PATIENT
SALUDO AL PACIENTE

Good morning. Good afternoon. Good evening.
Buenos días. Buenas tardes. Buenas noches.

(Mr./Mrs./Ms.) Gonzáles, how are you?
(Señor/Señora/Señorita) Gonzáles, ¿cómo está?

I'm glad you came.
Me alegro que haya venido.

Will you please sign in here?
¿Me haría el favor de firmar aquí?

Do you have your medical insurance card with you? Let me make a copy of it and then give it back to you.
¿Usted tiene su tarjeta de seguro médico consigo? Permítame hacerle una copia y después se la devuelvo.

Did you bring your completed "welcome to the office" form?
¿Usted trajo el formulario "bienvenido a nuestra oficina" completado?

Please fill out this form as completely as you can. It helps the doctor give you the best care possible. If you have any questions on how to fill it out, please let me know.
Por favor llene este formulario tan completamente como pueda. Esto ayuda al doctor proveerle el mejor cuidado posible.

Si tiene alguna pregunta de cómo llenarlo, por favor
déjeme saber.

I'll collect that completed form from you.
Voy a recolectar su formulario completado.

**Please have a seat in the reception area and make
yourself comfortable. I will need to enter your
information into our computer system.**
Por favor siéntese en el área de recepción y póngase cómodo.
Voy a tener que entrar su información en nuestro sistema de
computadora.

**One of our staff will call you back momentarily to
begin preliminary measurements before Dr. Castillo
sees you.**
Uno de los miembros de nuestro personal lo llamará
momentáneamente para comenzar las medidas preliminares
antes que el Dr. Castillo lo vea.

**Please turn off your cell phone while in the office so
that it does not interfere with our sensitive
instruments.**
Por favor apague su teléfono celular mientras esté en la oficina
para que éste no interfiera con nuestros instrumentos sensibles.

**My name is Carla. I am Dr. Castillo's assistant and will
be collecting additional information before you see
the doctor.**
Mi nombre es Carla. Yo soy la asistente del Dr. Castillo y estaré
recopilando información adicional antes que usted vea el doctor.

I'm Doctor Castillo. (Pass/Come) with me, please.
Yo soy el Doctor Castillo. (Pase/Venga) conmigo, por favor.

Welcome to our office. We will take good care of you.
Bienvenido a nuestra oficina. Voy a tomar buen cuidado de usted.

**You can leave your bag and other belongings here and
take a seat there.**
Usted puede dejar su bolsa y otras pertenencias aquí y tomar
asiento allá.

Chapter 2
Communicating and Courtesy

Capítulo 2
Comunicándose y Cortesía

UNDERSTANDING THE PATIENT
ENTENDER AL PACIENTE

Do you prefer to speak in Spanish or English?
¿Usted prefiere hablar en español o en inglés?

Excuse me? Please repeat what you told me.
¿Perdón? Por favor repita lo que me dijo.

**I didn't understand you completely. You told me
that ___ (fill in the blank), correct?**
No le entendí completamente. ¿Me dijo que ___ (fill in the
blank), correcto?

I still don't understand you.
Todavía no le entiendo.

**Can you please repeat what you said using different
words?**
¿Podría repetir lo que dijo usando palabras diferentes?

I still haven't learned the word.
Todavía no he aprendido la palabra.

I didn't understand anything you said to me.
No entendí nada de lo que me dijo.

**My Spanish is limited, and for that reason, speak to me
in (simple/common) words.**
Mi español es limitado, y por eso, hábleme con palabras
(sencillas/comunes).

Please speak more slowly.
Por favor hable más despacio.

I'm not familiar with that word.
No conozco esa palabra.

What is the (meaning/meaning) of that word?
¿Qué (significa/quiere decir) esa palabra?

I cannot hear you. Please speak louder.
No puedo oírle. Por favor, hable más fuerte.

I did not say that (to you).
No (le) dije eso.

I need a (translator/interpreter)—wait a minute.
Necesito un (traductor/intérprete)—espere un minuto.

MAKING SURE THE PATIENT UNDERSTANDS YOU
ASEGURARSE QUE EL PACIENTE LE ENTIENDE

Did you understand everything that I told you?
¿Entendió todo lo que le dije?

Do you have questions?
¿Tiene preguntas?

Do you have a question?
¿Tiene alguna pregunta?

EXPRESSING COURTESY
EXPRESAR CORTESÍA

Excuse me *(when getting in the way).* Excuse me *(when interrupting).* Pardon me.
Con permiso. Discúlpeme. Perdóneme.

I'm sorry *(e.g., expressing sympathy for death in the family).*
Lo siento.

I'm sorry you had to wait. We are very busy today.
Siento que haya tenido que esperar. Estamos muy
ocupados hoy.

Don't forget your bag.
No olvide su bolsa.

Take your time. Be careful!
Tome su tiempo. ¡Tenga cuidado!

One moment. My battery died.
Un momento. Mi batería murió.

Wait a minute—the battery (died/discharged).
Espere un minuto—la batería (se murió/se descargó).

**Please wait a minute. I need to get another
(bulb/Mexican for bulb).**
Espere un minuto, por favor. Necesito conseguir (otra
bombilla/otro foquito).

BIDDING FAREWELL
DESPEDIDA

Thank you very much.
Muchas gracias.

You're welcome. (It was nothing.)
De nada. (No fue nada.)

Don't mention it. (You're welcome.)
No hay de que.

I'm (very) happy to have served you.
Me da (mucho) gusto haberle atendido.

You are very kind.
Usted es muy amable.

Very nice knowing you (m./f.).
Mucho gusto en conocerlo/a.

Same to you.
Igualmente.

See you later.
Hasta luego.

Until next time. (See you soon.)
Hasta pronto.

Goodbye.
Adiós.

Capítulo 3
Tomando el Historial del Paciente

CHARACTERIZING GENERAL COMPLAINTS
CARACTERIZAR LAS QUEJAS GENERALES

What is the (purpose of your visit/reason for the exam) today?
¿Cuál es el (propósito de su visita/motivo del examen) hoy?

What is the reason for your visit?
¿Cuál es la razón de su visita?

How can I help you?
¿En qué puedo ayudarle?

Who sent you (m./f.) to me?
¿Quién (lo/la) mandó a mí?

Who (referred/sent) you (m./f.) to me?
¿Quién (lo/la) (refirió/mandó) a mí?

Who recommended us?
¿Quién nos recomendó?

Who referred you?
¿Quién le refirió?

For what reason?
¿Por qué razón?

Why?
¿Por qué?

How did you hear about us?
¿Cómo supo de nosotros?

Do you have a problem with your vision or eyes?
¿Tiene algún problema con su visión o sus ojos?

Do you have a specific problem?
¿Tiene algún problema específico?

Do you have any vision complaint?
¿Tiene alguna queja de la visión?

Have you noticed any change?
¿Ha notado algún cambio?

Have you noticed changes in your vision?
¿Ha notado cambios en su visión?

Have you noted changes in your vision since your last exam?
¿Ha tenido cambios en su visión desde su último examen?

Which eye, or are both affected?
¿En cuál ojo, o los dos están afectados?

Can you show me?
¿Puede mostrarme?

Can you show me?
¿Puede enseñarme?

Do you see well far away?
¿Usted ve bien de lejos?

Do you see well up close?
¿Usted ve bien de cerca?

When did this happen?
¿Cuándo le pasó esto?

When did it start?
¿Cuándo empezó esto?

Did it just start?
¿Apenas empezó?

Was the change sudden or (gradual/progressive)?
¿El cambio fue de repente o (poco a poco/progresivo)?

Did you lose your vision gradually?
¿Usted perdió la visión poco a poco?

How often have you had this problem?
¿Cuántas veces ha tenido este problema?

Do you have it (all the time/almost always/once in a while/almost never)?
¿Usted lo tiene (todo el tiempo/casi siempre/de vez en cuando/casi nunca)?

How long (does it last/did it last)?
¿Cuánto tiempo (le dura/le duró)?

Tell me, where does it hurt?
Dígame, ¿dónde le duele?

Has your pain gone away?
¿Se le quitó el dolor?

How long have you had it?
¿Por cuánto tiempo lo ha tenido?

How long have you had it?
¿Cuánto tiempo hace que lo tiene?

Since when have you had this problem?
¿Desde cuándo tiene este problema?

When was the last time it happened?
¿Cuándo fue la última vez que ocurrió?

How much do your eyes bother you?
¿Qué tanto le molestan sus ojos?

How much does it irritate you?
¿Cuánto le irrita?

How much is the irritation?
¿Cuánta es la molestia?

What do you do to relieve the irritation?
¿Qué usted hace para aliviar la irritación?

Do your eyes feel well?
¿Se sienten bien sus ojos?

How do your eyes feel?
¿Cómo siente sus ojos?

SPECIFIC COMPLAINTS
QUEJAS ESPECÍFICAS

Do you feel something in your eye?
¿Usted siente algo en su ojo?

Do your eyes get red?
¿Se ponen rojos sus ojos?

Do you wake up with discharge (Mexican/Guatemalan) in your eyes?
¿Amanece con (lagañas/chelo) en sus ojos?

Do you have difficulty seeing at night?
¿Tiene dificultad para ver de noche?

Does the sun bother you a lot?
¿Le molesta mucho el sol?

Are you very sensitive to intense light?
¿Es usted muy sensible a la luz intensa?

Do you see cobwebs in your vision?
¿Usted ve telarañas en su visión?

Do you see little lights or spots?
¿Usted ve lucecitas o manchas?

Did a stick penetrate your eye?
¿Penetró una vara su ojo?

Do you think it is a (small piece/burr) of wood or metal?
¿Piensa usted que es (un pedacito/una rebaba) de madera o metal?

Do your eyes feel very dry?
¿Sus ojos se sienten muy resecos?

Do your eyes feel dry?
¿Sus ojos se sienten resecos?

Do you (suffer/suffer) from (itch/itch)?
¿(Padece/Sufre) de (comezón/picazón)?

Do you have eye mucous discharge?
¿Sus ojos tienen lagañas?

Do your eyes burn or hurt?
¿Le arden o le duelen sus ojos?

Do you suffer from headaches while using your eyes?
¿Usted sufre de dolores de cabeza mientras usa sus ojos?

Where does it hurt?
¿Dónde le duele?

What are you doing when it hurts?
¿Qué está haciendo cuando le duele?

Are you reading much when it hurts?
¿Usted está leyendo mucho cuando le duele?

When you read a lot, does it hurt?
Cuando lee mucho, ¿le duele?

Are you not reading because you can't see or because you don't want to?
¿No está leyendo porque no puede ver o porque no quiere?

Have you ever seen double?
¿Ha visto doble alguna vez?

Are you seeing things double right now?
¿Ve las cosas doble ahora mismo?

I need to perform some tests to make sure this is the reason.
Necesito hacer unas pruebas para asegurar que ésta es la razón.

SOCIAL HISTORY
ANTECEDENTES SOCIALES

What is your name?
¿Cómo se llama?

Where were you born?
¿Dónde nació?

What is your address?
¿Cuál es su dirección?

Where are you from?
¿De dónde es?

How old are you?
¿Cuántos años tiene usted?

What is your birthdate?
¿Cuál es su fecha de nacimiento?

Are you working?
¿Está trabajando?

What do you do for work?
¿En qué está trabajando?

Are you a housewife?
¿Es usted ama de casa?

What is the name of your employer or company?
¿Cuál es el nombre de su patrón o compañía?

Your telephone (number) please? And your number where you work?
¿Su número de teléfono, por favor? ¿Y el número de teléfono de donde trabaja?

Do you work on a computer?
¿Trabaja usted con una computadora?

How many hours do you work each day on a computer?
¿Cuántas horas al día usted trabaja con una computadora?

Does your work involve grinding metal, hammering, or other activities which may cause particles to get into your eye?
¿Su trabajo envuelve amolar metal, martillar u otras actividades que pueden hacer que le caigan partículas en su ojo?

Does your work require you to wear safety glasses?
¿Su trabajo requiere que use lentes de seguridad?

Do you have kids?
¿Usted tiene niños?

Do the kids cause trouble?
¿Los niños hacen travesuras?

What do you do with your free time?
¿Qué le gusta hacer con su tiempo libre?

What sports and hobbies do you do?
¿Qué deportes y pasatiempos practica?

Do you drink much alcohol?
¿Usted bebe mucho alcohol?

Do you smoke?
¿Usted fuma?

LAST EYE EXAM
ÚLTIMO EXAMEN DE LA VISTA

Is this your first eye exam?
¿Es éste su primer examen de la vista?

When was your last eye exam?
¿Cuándo fue su último examen de la vista?

Did everything go well?
¿Todo salió bien?

Have your eyes been dilated before?
¿Sus ojos han sido dilatados alguna vez?

Did the doctors tell you that you have an eye disease?
¿Los doctores le dijeron que usted tiene una enfermedad de los ojos?

What did the doctors tell you?
¿Qué le dijeron los doctores?

LAST PRESCRIPTION
ÚLTIMA RECETA

How old are your glasses?
¿Qué tan viejos son sus anteojos?

How old are your current glasses?
¿Cuánto tiempo tienen sus anteojos actuales?

How are you doing with your glasses?
¿Cómo le va con los anteojos?

Do they still work well?
¿Todavía le sirven bien?

Are your glasses broken?
¿Sus anteojos están (quebrados/rotos)?

Are your glasses worn down?
¿Sus anteojos están desgastados?

Are your glasses scratched?
¿Sus anteojos están (raspados/rayados)?

Are your glasses lost?
¿Sus anteojos están perdidos?

Did you (lose/misplace) your glasses?
¿Se le (perdieron/extraviaron) los anteojos?

Did you bring your glasses?
¿Trajo sus anteojos?

Get them please.
Consígalos, por favor.

Have you used contact lenses (*formal/informal*)?
¿Ha usado (lentes de contacto/lentes de pupila)?

CONTACT LENS HISTORY
ANTECEDENTES DE LENTES DE CONTACTO

Have you used contact lenses before?
¿Usted ha usado lentes de contacto anteriormente?

Are you now using contact lenses?
¿Usted usa ahora lentes de contacto?

Are you interested in contact lenses?
¿Está usted interesado/a en lentes de contacto?

What care system do you use for the lenses—for example, "OptiFree Express" or "Renu"?
¿Qué sistema de cuidado de lentes usted usa—por ejemplo, "OptiFree Express" o "Renu"?

How many days during the week do you sleep with your contact lenses?
¿Cuántos días durante la semana duerme con sus lentes de contacto?

Are they hard or soft?
¿Son rígidos o blandos?

Are they disposable?
¿Son desechables?

Have you used contact lenses in the past?
¿Usted ha usado lentes de contacto en el pasado?

Why did you stop using them?
¿Por qué dejó de usarlos?

Do you know the brand of the contact lenses?
¿Usted sabe la marca de los lentes de contacto?

How old are the lenses that you're using?
¿Qué tan viejos son los lentes que está usando?

How comfortable are your lenses?
¿Qué tan cómodos son sus lentes?

How is your vision with your lenses?
¿Cómo está su visión con sus lentes?

Normally, at what hour do you put them in and take them out?
Normalmente, ¿a qué hora se los pone y se los quita?

Approximately how long do you use your contact lenses every day?
Aproximadamente, ¿por cuánto tiempo se pone sus lentes de contacto cada día?

PAST OCULAR HISTORY
ANTECEDENTES OCULARES PASADOS

In the past, did you ever injure your eyes?
En el pasado, ¿alguna vez se ha lastimado sus ojos?

Did your eye suffer any trauma?
¿Su ojo sufrió algún golpe?

Did your eye receive any trauma?
¿Es ojo sufrió algún golpe?

Do you know if you have any eye disease, for example, glaucoma?
¿Usted sabe si tiene alguna enfermedad de los ojos, por ejemplo glaucoma?

Have you had surgery or infections of the eyes?
¿Ha tenido cirugía o infecciones de los ojos?

How did you lose this eye? What happened?
¿Cómo perdió este ojo? ¿Qué pasó?

PERSONAL MEDICAL HISTORY
ANTECEDENTES MÉDICOS PERSONALES

How is your general health?
¿Cómo está su salud general?

When was your last physical exam?
¿Cuándo fue su último examen físico?

Who is your primary care doctor?
¿Quién es su médico principal?

Are you pregnant? Congratulations!
¿Está embarazada? ¡Felicidades!

Do you have high blood pressure, diabetes, or thyroid problems?
¿Usted tiene alta presión sanguínea, diabetes o problemas de la tiroides?

Do you know if your diabetes is type I or II (or gestational)?
¿Sabe si su diabetes es tipo uno o dos (o de embarazo)?

More recently, how was your blood sugar level?
Más recientemente, ¿cómo fue su nivel de azúcar en la sangre?

Did you have a stroke?
¿Usted tuvo una apoplejía?

MEDICATIONS AND ALLERGIES
MEDICAMENTOS Y ALERGIAS

Do you have allergies?
¿Usted tiene alergias?

Are you allergic (m./f.) to any medicines?
¿Es alérgico/a a alguna medicina?

Is all the medicine finished?
¿Se le terminó toda la medicina?

Do you want to refill the medicine?
¿Quiere volver a surtir la medicina?

You are not using any kind of (eye) drops?
¿No está usando ninguna clase de gotas para los ojos?

How many times a day?
¿Cuántas veces al día?

Chapter 4
Visual Acuity

Capítulo 4
Agudeza Visual

PREPARATION
PREPARACIÓN

Description to patient: **I will be evaluating how well each of your eyes sees on a letter chart.**
Voy a estar evaluando cuán bien cada uno de sus ojos ve con un letrero de letras.

Stand here.
Párese aquí.

Move a bit to your right/left.
Muévase un poco hacia su derecha/izquierda.

Do you know how to read?
¿Usted sabe leer?

Can you put the glasses on? Can you take off the glasses?
¿Puede ponerse los anteojos? ¿Puede quitarse los anteojos?

Can you put them on? Can you take them off?
¿Puede ponérselos? ¿Puede quitárselos?

Put them on, please. Take them off, please.
Póngaselos, por favor. Quíteselos, por favor.

Cover your (left/right) eye. Cover your other eye.
Cubra su ojo (izquierdo/derecho). Cubra su otro ojo.

Keep that eye covered.
Mantenga ese ojo cubierto.

Don't squint.
No entrecierre sus ojos.

Don't move forward.
No se mueva hacia delante.

MEASUREMENT
MEDIDAS

How many fingers do I have?
¿Cuántos dedos tengo?

Can you see my hand moving?
¿Puede ver mi mano moviéndose?

Can you see the light? Where?
¿Puede ver la luz? ¿Dónde?

To what line can you see?
¿Hasta cuál línea puede ver?

Can you see to the bottommost?
¿Puede ver hasta la de más abajo?

Can you see to the last line?
¿Puede ver hasta la última línea?

What are these letters?
¿Cuáles son esas letras?

Read me this line. And the next. And below this one?
  (Continue/continue.)
Léame esta línea. Y la próxima. ¿Y abajo de ésa? (Siga/continúe.)

Read from top to bottom. Do the best you can.
Lea de arriba hacia abajo. Haga lo mejor que pueda.

You don't see them?
¿No las ve?

Tell me something. Read them now.
Dígame algo. Léalas ahora.

Tell me the smallest one you can read. You can guess.
Dígame las más pequeñas que puede leer. Puede adivinar.

Begin with the letter "T".
Comience con la letra "T".

These letters are extra. Most people can't read those.
Estas letras son adicionales. La mayoría de las personas no pueden leer esas.

Those letters are very small. Few can read them.
Esas letras son muy pequeñas. Pocos pueden leerlas.

Can you make them out?
¿Las puede distinguir?

You can't distinguish them well?
¿No las distingue bien?

Look at the very last line.
Mire la última línea de abajo.

Can't see it?
¿No la puede ver?

Can hardly see them?
¿Apenas las ve?

Is it (blurry/clear)?
¿Está (borroso/claro)?

PINHOLE ACUITY
AGUDEZA DE AGUJERO

Now look through these pinholes.
Ahora, mire por los agujeros.

You have to move the pinhole just right to get the best vision.
Usted tiene que mover el agujero precisamente para tener la mejor visión.

Do they help you?
¿Ellos le ayudan?

EYE CHARTS FOR THE ILLITERATE
LETREROS PARA LOS ANALFABETOS

Point to character on "tumbling E" chart: **Where are the legs of the letter going?**
¿Adónde van las patitas de la letra?

Show me, up like this, down, this side, or the other side?
Muéstreme, ¿para arriba así, abajo, este lado o el otro lado?

How about now?
¿Y ahora?

Point to character on Allen or Lea chart: **What is this?**
¿Qué es esto?

A (duck/chicken/bird)?
¿(Un pato/Una gallina/Un pájaro)?

A (pastry/cake/sponge cake)?
¿(Un pastel/Una torta/Un bizcocho)?

A hand?
¿Una mano?

A (car/car/automobile)?
¿Un (carro/coche/automóvil)?

A telephone?
¿Un teléfono?

A horse?
¿Un caballo?

A heart?
¿Un corazón?

An apple?
¿Una manzana?

A circle?
¿Un círculo?

A square?
¿Un cuadrado?

A house?
¿Una casa?

DIRECT, CONSENSUAL, AND MARCUS-GUNN TESTING
EXAMINACIÓN DIRECTA, CONSENSUAL Y MARCUS-GUNN

Description to patient: **I will now perform some measurements of the nerve function of your eyes.**
Ahora voy a tomar algunas medidas de la función nerviosa de sus ojos.

Look ahead. I have a bright light for examining the pupil reflexes. Don't look at my light.
Mire hacia adelante. Tengo una luz brillante para examinar los reflejos pupilares. No mire mi luz.

Your pupil reflexes are normal.
Sus reflejos pupilares son normales.

BRIGHTNESS COMPARISON
COMPARACIÓN DE INTENSIDAD DE LUZ

Showing light monocularly: **If the brightness of this light is worth one hundred pesos with this eye, how much is it worth with the other?**
¿Si la intensidad de esta luz vale cien pesos con este ojo, cuánto vale con el otro?

RED DESATURATION
DESATURACIÓN DEL ROJO

What color is the cap of this bottle?
¿De qué color es el tapón de esta botella?

With this eye, do you see the same level of redness?
¿Con este ojo, usted ve el mismo nivel de rojo?

Is it pink?
¿Es rosa?

Chapter 6
Directing Gaze for Cover Test, Versions, Retinoscopy, Slit Lamp, and Fundoscopy

Capítulo 6
Dirigiendo la Mirada para el Examen Cubierto, las Versiones, la Retinoscopia, Lámpara de Abertura, y Oftalmoscopia

(Look/Find) the letter chart in the mirror.
(Mire/Busque) el letrero en el espejo.

You don't have to tell me the letters.
No tiene que decirme las letras.

Fixate on the big "E" and keep it clear.
Fíjese en la letra "E" grande y manténgala clara.

Follow the light only with your eyes. Now, try to follow it to your nose.
Siga la luz solamente con sus ojos. Ahora, trate de seguirla hasta su nariz.

Keep looking at one point and don't move your eyes.
Siga mirando en un punto y no mueva sus ojos.

You are moving your eyes too much. You can still blink, but keep your eyes pointed at this knob.
Está moviendo sus ojos demasiado. Puede parpadear, pero mantenga sus ojos enfocados en esta perilla.

The whole time, keep looking at the red and green.
En todo momento, siga mirando el rojo y el verde.

Look past my ear toward the wall.
Mire más allá de mi oreja hacia la pared.

Look toward the right, the left, up, down——without moving your head.
Mire hacia la derecha, la izquierda, arriba, abajo—sin mover la cabeza.

Look (forward/straight ahead/straight ahead).
Mire (adelante/derecho/al frente).

Description to patient: **I will now measure your ability to see depth perception using the two eyes.**
Ahora voy a medir su habilidad de ver percepción de profundidad usando los dos ojos.

Please put on these special glasses over your existing reading glasses.
Por favor póngase estos anteojos especiales sobre sus anteojos de leer existentes.

Which of these (animals/circles) is jumping out of the box?
¿Cuál de estos (animales/círculos) está saltando fuera del cuadro?

How about the next one?
¿Qué tal el próximo?

It gets harder and harder. Can you guess?
Se vuelve más y más difícil. ¿Puede adivinar?

Starting with number one, which of the three circles seems different or appears to stand out in front of the other two?
Comenzando con el número uno, ¿cuál de estos tres círculos se ve diferente o parece sobresalir al frente de los otros dos?

Tell me, is it the left, middle, or right circle?
Dígame, ¿es el círculo de la izquierda, el del centro o el de la derecha?

How about number two, three, four, etc.?
¿Qué tal el número dos, tres, cuatro, etc.?

Please do not move the test book any closer, or else you may throw off an accurate measurement.
Por favor no mueva el libro de prueba más cerca, o podría hacer perder una medida precisa.

Chapter 8
Color Vision (Pseudoisochromatic and D-15)

Capítulo 8
Visión en Color (Seudoisocromática y D-15)

Description to patient: **Let's see how well you can distinguish colors.**
Veamos cuán bien usted puede distinguir los colores.

This is a test of color vision.
Ésta es una prueba para la visión de colores.

This test is for knowing whether you correctly perceive colors.
Esta prueba es para saber si percibe correctamente los colores.

What number do you see? What is it?
¿Qué número ve? ¿Cuál es?

It is OK if you have trouble and don't see anything.
Está bien si tiene problemas y no ve nada.

Can you see a number here?
¿Puede ver un número aquí?

Pointing to D-15 color caps: **Put these things in order according to similar colors.** *Point to first cap:* **Begin with this.**
Ponga estas cosas en orden según colores similares. Empiece con ésta.

Please don't touch the colored part of the cap or plate. Oils and dirt from the fingers cause the hues to discolor over time.

Por favor no toque la parte coloreada del tapón o el plato. Los aceites y el sucio de los dedos causa que los colores se destinten con el tiempo.

You have normal color vision.
Usted tiene una visión de color normal.

You have a color deficiency. This is relatively common. About 6 to 8 percent of males have a color deficiency. Even though you still perceive colors, there will be certain hues which you may confuse with one another even though you won't even know it.
Usted tiene una deficiencia de color. Esto es relativamente común. Alrededor de un 6 a 8 por ciento de los varones tiene deficiencia de color. Aunque usted sí percibe los colores, hay ciertos colores que usted puede confundir con otros aunque usted ni siquiera lo sabrá.

Color deficiency is different from color blindness, an extremely rare condition in which those affected see only in black and white. Although color deficiency usually won't affect your day-to-day life, it can limit your occupational choices. Normal color vision is generally necessary to become a policeman, firefighter, electrician, and pilot.
La deficiencia de color es diferente al daltonismo, una condición extremadamente rara en la cual los afectados sólo ven en blanco y negro. Aunque la deficiencia de color generalmente no afectará su vida diaria, puede limitar sus opciones ocupacionales. La visión de color normal es necesaria para ser un policía, bombero, electricista y piloto.

Chapter 9
Positioning the Patient for Keratometry, Corneal Topography, Slit Lamp, Refraction, Binocular Indirect Ophthalmoscopy, and Drop Instillation

Capítulo 9
Posicionando al Paciente para la Queratometría, Topografía de la Cornea, Lámpara de Abertura, Refracción, Oftalmoscopia Binocular Indirecta, e Instilación de Gotas

Now it's your turn.
Ahora le toca a usted.

It's your turn.
Es su turno.

You're next.
Usted sigue.

Come on over and have a seat in the examination chair.
Venga y siéntese en la silla de examen.

Sit straight. Sit comfortably. Loosen up/relax.
Siéntese (recto/derecho). Siéntese cómodamente. Relájese.

Can you take off your hat?
¿Puede quitarse su sombrero?

Stand up for a moment. I want to adjust your seat.
Párese un momento. Quiero ajustar el asiento.

Come closer. Bring your forehead up against the plastic.
Acérquese. Arrime su frente contra el plástico.

I'm going to raise you (m./f.) up higher.
(Lo/La) voy a subir más alto.

Keep your forehead against the plastic bar.
Mantenga su frente contra la barra de plástico.

Put your chin here and your forehead up here.
Ponga su barbilla aquí y la frente acá arriba.

Keep looking ahead in the center of the tube.
Siga mirando adelante por el centro del tubo.

Don't get so close because your breath is fogging the lenses.
No se arrime tan cerca porque su aliento está empañando los lentes.

Put your hair back.
Eche su pelo hacia atrás.

Open your eyes really wide.
Abra sus ojos bien grandes.

Don't hold your breath. Just breath normally.
No aguante la respiración. Sólo respire normalmente.

Blink as you like. Relax (your eyes/eyelids).
Parpadee a su gusto. Relaje sus (ojos/párpados).

Look at the tips of my fingers and keep your eyes in this direction.
Mire a las puntas de mis dedos y mantenga sus ojos en esta dirección.

A little bit higher, lower, right, left. Perfect.
Un poquito más alto, más abajo, más a la derecha, más a la izquierda. Perfecto.

(Raise/lower) the chin.
(Levante/baje) la barbilla.

I'm going to flip the eyelid. Keep looking down.
Le voy a voltear el párpado. Siga mirando hacia abajo.

No, it does not hurt, although it'll feel funny.
No, no duele, aunque se sentirá raro.

Chapter 10
Visual Fields

Capítulo 10
Campos Visuales

Description to patient: **I will now evaluate your peripheral vision. Side vision problems can signal damage inside the eye or even within the brain. Conditions that reduce peripheral vision include glaucoma and other diseases of the optic nerve.**

Ahora voy a evaluar su visión periférica. Los problemas de visión lateral pueden indicar daños dentro del ojo o hasta en el cerebro. Las condiciones que reducen la visión periférica incluyen el glaucoma y otras enfermedades del nervio óptico.

FINGER COUNTING
CONTEO DE DEDOS

Cover this eye and keep looking in the center of my open eye.

Cubra este ojo y siga mirando en el centro de mi ojo abierto.

With your peripheral vision, how many fingers are there in total?

Con su visión periférica, ¿cuántos dedos hay en total?

Remember to keep your eye pointed right here. If your eye wanders, I cannot properly evaluate your side vision.

Acuérdese de mantener su ojo dirigido hacia aquí. Si su ojo se mueve, no puedo evaluar correctamente su visión lateral.

AUTOMATED-HUMPHREY VISUAL FIELD
CAMPO VISUAL HUMPHREY AUTOMATIZADO

This is a test of your peripheral vision.
Ésta es una prueba de su visión periférica.

Consequently, it is important that you keep looking at the main light, in the center all the time.
Por eso, es importante que usted siga mirando la luz principal en el centro, todo el tiempo.

If you think there is a light in your peripheral vision, press the button.
Si usted cree que hay una luz en su visión periférica, oprima el botón.

Do not move your eye during the test. Keep looking in the center.
No mueva su ojo durante la prueba. Siga mirando al centro.

You finished half of it.
Ya terminó la mitad.

FREQUENCY DOUBLING TECHNOLOGY (FDT) VISUAL FIELD
CAMPO VISUAL POR TECNOLOGÍA DE DUPLICACIÓN DE FRECUENCIA

During the test, always keep looking in the center at the little black square.
Durante la prueba, siempre mire al centro al cuadrito negro.

If you think there are lines moving in your peripheral vision, press the button.
Si usted cree que hay líneas moviéndose en su visión periférica, oprima el botón.

The test lasts less than one minute.
La prueba dura menos de un minuto.

It is like a video game.
Es como un juego de video.

You can blink, but it is important that you don't move your eyes around.
Usted puede parpadear, pero es importante que no mueva sus ojos.

Ready (m./f.)? We are going to begin right now.
¿Listo/a? Vamos a empezar ahora mismo.

If you see the wiggly lines, go ahead and click the button.
Si ve las líneas onduladas, oprima el botón.

Don't move your eye around. Keep it pointed straight ahead.
No mueva su ojo. Manténgalo dirigido hacia delante.

You are clicking the button even when the visual stimulus is not shown. Do you understand this measurement? You should click the button only if you see the wiggly lines.
Usted está oprimiendo el botón aún cuando no se está mostrando el estímulo visual. ¿Usted entiende esta prueba? Debería oprimir el botón sólo si usted ve las líneas onduladas.

All right, let's move on to your other eye.
Muy bien, sigamos con su otro ojo.

AMSLER GRID
CUADRÍCULA DE AMSLER

Handing patient Amsler grid: **Take this lined table, like this.**
Sujete esta tabla con líneas, así.

Always keep your gaze at the center of the table.
Siempre mantenga su vista en el centro de la tabla.

Don't move it any closer or further away.
No la mueva más cerca o más lejos.

With your peripheral vision, do you see all the corners?
¿Con su visión periférica, ve todas las esquinas?

Are some parts of the table distorted or missing?
¿Hay algunas partes de la tabla que están distorsionadas o que
   faltan?

Show me.
Muéstreme.

Chapter 11
Retinoscopy

Capítulo 11
Retinoscopia

Description to patient: **By shining a light using a special instrument, I can get a rough idea of how well your eyes bring objects into focus and what type of glasses prescription you may need. This technique is how glasses are often prescribed for non-verbal children.**

Iluminando con una luz usando un instrumento especial, puedo tener una idea aproximada de cuán bien sus ojos enfocan sobre los objetos y qué tipo de receta de anteojos puede necesitar. Esta técnica es cómo se recetan anteojos a los niños que no hablan.

Don't look at my light. Keep looking far away in the direction of the eye chart.

No mire mi luz. Siga mirando a lo lejos en la dirección del letrero.

I am focusing light at the back of the eye.

Estoy enfocando la luz en el fondo del ojo.

Don't worry if you see everything blurry.

No se preocupe si usted ve todo borroso.

I will clear things up momentarily.

Voy a aclarar las cosas momentáneamente.

Chapter 12
Refraction-Binocular Humphriss

Capítulo 12
Refracción-Binocular de Humphriss

Right now, your right eye is clearer than the other, correct?
Ahora mismo, ¿el ojo derecho es más claro que el otro, correcto?

Still, keep both eyes open.
Todavía, mantenga los dos ojos abiertos.

Look at the small ones. Look carefully.
Mire a las pequeñas. Mire con cuidado.

And is this better or worse?
¿Y éste es mejor o peor?

Are the letters clearer or blurrier now?
¿Las letras están más claras o más borrosas ahora?

Are the two equal?
¿Los dos son iguales?

The same?
¿Lo mismo?

Equally (clear/ugly) this one?
Este, ¿igual de (claro/feo)?

You don't see any difference?
¿No ve ninguna diferencia?

Between lens one and two, which is better?

Entre el lente uno y el dos, ¿cuál es mejor?

Which lens do you see better with, lens one or lens two?

¿Con cuál lente ve mejor, el lente uno o el lente dos?

Better this one or the second?

¿Mejor éste o el segundo?

Which is better, one or two?

¿Cuál es mejor, uno o dos?

Better one … or two?

¿Mejor uno … o dos?

Was the one before better?

¿El anterior era mejor?

Both can't be better, only one. Look again carefully.

Los dos no pueden estar mejor, solamente uno. Mire con cuidado otra vez.

Yes, both are almost the same. But better or worse here?

Sí, los dos son casi iguales. ¿Pero mejor o peor aquí?

The two are going to be blurry. But of the two ways, which lens is better?

Los dos van a estar borrosos. Pero de las dos maneras, ¿cuál lente es mejor?

I'm only interested if it's better or worse.

Solamente me interesa si es mejor o peor.

Is this better?

¿Éste es mejor?

Do you prefer this one?

¿Prefiere éste?

Are the letters better here?
¿Están mejor las letras así?

Is this one more comfortable?
¿Éste es más cómodo?

A little bit worse here?
¿Un poco peor acá?

A little better or worse now?
¿Un poco mejor o peor ahora?

Does this make it worse?
¿Esto lo hace peor?

Did the letters become blurry?
¿Se pusieron borrosas las letras?

Well blurred here?
¿Bien borrosas aquí?

Are they blurred?
¿Están empañadas?

Blurrier?
¿Más borrosas?

Tell me when you don't see the letters well.
Dígame cuando ya no vea bien las letras.

Are you sure (m./f.)?
¿Éstá seguro/a?

Box 12-1. Common patient comments during refraction	Cuadro 12-1. Comentarios comunes de los pacientes durante la refracción
I can't see any of the letters.	No puedo ver ninguna de las letras.
Everything is blurry.	Todo está borroso.
Can you show me the lenses again?	¿Puede mostrarme los lentes otra vez?
Lens one is distorted up and down, and in lens two the letters are distorted another way.	El lente uno está distorsionado hacia arriba y abajo, y en el lente dos las letras están distorsionadas de otra manera.
Both look the same.	Los dos se ven iguales.
I can't see anything else.	No puedo ver nada más.
I can barely see those letters.	Casi no puedo ver esas letras.

Chapter 13
Near Testing with Relative Accommodation, Binocular Cross-Cylinder, and Free-Space Trial

Capítulo 13
Examen de Cerca con Acomodación Relativa, Cilindro Cruzado Binocular, y Prueba de Espacio Libre

Now, I'm going to do a few tests for close-up vision.
Ahora, voy a hacer unas cuantas pruebas para la visión de cerca.

Tell me when these letters start to (blur/clear).
Dígame cuando esas letras empiezan a (borrarse/aclararse).

Are they still clear?
¿Todavía están claras?

Once again, the same thing.
Otra vez, la misma cosa.

This is a cross with lines (going side to side/going side to side) and up and down.
Ésa es una cruz con líneas (acostadas/atravesadas) y paradas.

Right now, the ones lying down are darkest, correct?
¿Ahora, las acostadas están más oscuras, correcto?

Tell me when the others are the darkest and most distinct.
Dígame cuando las otras sean las más oscuras y más distinguibles.

Can you focus and make them clear?
¿Puede enfocar y hacerlas claras?

Hold this card.
Sujete esta tarjeta.

Give me this card.
Déme esta tarjeta.

I am going to hold some lenses over your old glasses. Does this help you?
Voy a sostener unos lentes sobre sus anteojos viejos. ¿Esto le ayuda?

What I showed you was the change in your glasses prescription.
Lo que le mostré fue el cambio en la receta de sus anteojos.

You definitely need new glasses!
¡Usted definitivamente necesita anteojos nuevos!

Chapter 14
Tonometry (Goldmann and Non-Contact)

Capítulo 14
Tonometría (Goldmann y sin contacto)

Description to patient: **I will now perform a simple measurement that indirectly measures the fluid pressure in the eye. This is useful for the doctor to diagnose conditions including glaucoma.**

Ahora voy a hacer unas medidas simples que miden indirectamente la presión de líquido en el ojo. Esto es útil para que el doctor diagnostique condiciones incluyendo el glaucoma.

DROP INSTILLATION
INSTILACIÓN DE GOTAS

This is a tissue for the drops.
Ésta es una toallita para las gotas.

I (will "pour" you/will put) a drop in each eye.
(Le echaré/Voy a poner) una gota en cada ojo.

This is some anesthetic. I'm going to put some yellow color in the tears.
Esto es un poco de anestesia. Voy a poner un poco de color amarillo en las lágrimas.

Tip your head back.
Incline la cabeza hacia atrás.

It's possible the drops may sting a bit. Keep your eyes closed for a while.
Es posible que las gotas ardan un poco. Mantenga sus ojos cerrados por un rato.

Now you can dry your eyes. It wasn't too bad, right?
Ya se puede secar sus ojos. ¿No fue tan mal, verdad?

PROCEDURE
PROCEDIMIENTO

This blue light will come close to your eyelashes.
Esta luz azul se va a acercar a sus pestañas.

Open your eyes wide and don't blink for five seconds.
Abra sus ojos bien grandes y no parpadee por cinco segundos.

In just a moment, you will feel a puff of air.
En un momento sentirá un soplo de aire.

Don't squeeze your eyelids.
No apriete sus párpados.

Please try to relax your eyelids.
Por favor, trate de relajar sus párpados.

Chapter 15
Gonioscopy and Contact Lens Fundoscopy

Capítulo 15
Gonioscopía y Oftalmoscopia con Lentes de Contacto

I'm going to apply a special contact lens on your eye to examine it better.

Voy a poner un lente de contacto especial sobre su ojo para examinarlo mejor.

It may feel strange but it won't hurt you. It feels like an eye under water.

Se puede sentir extraño pero no le hará daño. Se siente como un ojo bajo agua.

This special lens allows me to evaluate the part of the eye where internal fluid drains out.

Este lente especial me permite evaluar la parte del ojo donde se drena el líquido interno.

In some patients, the fluid drain becomes clogged with debris or can be diseased.

En algunos pacientes, el drenaje de líquido se tapa con desechos o puede estar enfermo.

This special lens allows me to clearly evaluate the fine detail of the retina.

Este lente especial me permite evaluar claramente el detalle fino de la retina.

Chapter 16
Dilation Drops

Capítulo 16
Gotas para la Dilatación

EXPLANATION
EXPLICACIÓN

These drops are for dilating the pupils (*formal/informal*) of the eyes.
Estas gotas son para dilatar las (pupilas/niñas) de los ojos.

The drops make the pupils large and relax their ability to focus.
Las gotas hacen las pupilas bien grandes y relajan su habilidad de enfocar.

The dilated exam will cost fifty dollars more.
El examen de dilatación costará cincuenta dólares más.

It is important, because without the drops, it is hard to determine if there are problems inside.
Es importante, porque sin las gotas, es difícil determinar si hay problemas adentro.

It is very important that you have the dilation to determine the eye's state of health.
Es muy importante que tenga la dilatación para determinar el estado de salud del ojo.

There are many types of diseases that frequently exist without symptoms.
Hay bastantes tipos de enfermedades que existen con frecuencia sin síntomas.

A dilated exam is crucial for determining if there are problems at the back of the eye.
Un examen dilatado es crucial para determinar si hay problemas en la parte de atrás del ojo.

There are problems such as glaucoma, cataracts, retinal detachment, or holes in the retina.
Hay problemas como glaucoma, cataratas, retina desprendida o agujeros en la retina.

If you don't want the drops today, I can dilate the pupils when you pick up your glasses.
Si no quiere las gotas hoy, puedo dilatar las pupilas cuando recoja sus anteojos.

FOLLOWING INSTILLATION
DESPUÉS DE LA INSTILACIÓN

In twenty minutes, give or take, the eyes will feel the effect of the medicine.
En veinte minutos, más o menos, los ojos van a sentir el efecto de la medicina.

Meanwhile, let's go choose your new glasses.
Mientras tanto, vamos a escoger sus anteojos nuevos.

Meanwhile, you'll need to wait outside on the (bench/chair/sofa).
Mientras tanto, tendrá que esperar afuera en (la banca/la silla/ el sofá).

Come with me. Follow me, please.
Venga conmigo. Sígame, por favor.

Your pupils will remain enlarged for several hours before they return to normal. Meanwhile, you may find it difficult to read and lights will seem unusually bright.
Sus pupilas permanecerán engrandecidas por varias horas antes de regresar a lo normal. Mientras tanto, se le puede hacer difícil leer y las luces pueden parecer muy intensas.

Here are some disposable sunglasses for you to wear over your distance glasses.
Aquí tiene unos lentes de sol desechables para que las use sobre sus anteojos de distancia.

You should be able to comfortably drive home with sunglasses. However, if you do not feel comfortable, please wait until your vision returns to a level you feel comfortable driving home with.
Usted debería ser capaz de manejar cómodamente hasta su casa con los lentes de sol. Sin embargo, si no se siente cómodo, por favor espere hasta que su visión regrese a un nivel que usted siente es cómodo para manejar hasta su casa.

If you'd like, I can instill an eye drop that speeds up the recovery from the dilation by about half the usual time. However, it stings on instillation and it will make your eyes red for about 45 minutes. Would you like me to instill the reversal drop?
Si quiere, puedo poner una gota en el ojo que acelera la recuperación de la dilatación por la mitad del tiempo usual. Sin embargo, arde al echarlas y hará sus ojos rojos por alrededor de 45 minutos. ¿Le gustaría que le ponga la gota de inversión?

Chapter 17
Binocular Indirect Ophthalmoscopy

Capítulo 17
Oftalmoscopia Indirecta Binocular

GENERAL
GENERAL

Now, I'm going to look inside your eyes.
Ahora, voy a mirar dentro de sus ojos.

Did the light dazzle you? I'm sorry, the light is very strong.
¿Le encandiló la luz? Discúlpeme, la luz es muy fuerte.

Look up, up and to the right, right, down and to the right, down, down and to the left, left, up and to the left.
Mire para arriba, arriba y a la derecha, a la derecha, abajo y a la derecha, abajo, abajo y a la izquierda, a la izquierda, arriba y a la izquierda.

As I shine the light around, you may notice the shadows of some of the blood vessels in your eye. They look like tree branches.
Mientras muevo la luz, usted puede notar las sombras de algunos de los vasos sanguíneos en su ojo. Parecen ramas de árboles.

SCLERAL INDENTATION
HENDIDURA ESCLERAL

I'm going to put a bit of pressure on the eyelid, like this (*apply pressure*), in order to see the retina better.
Voy a poner un poco de presión sobre el párpado, así, para mirar la retina mejor.

By applying pressure, I am able to push some of the edges of the retina into my field of view.
Al aplicar presión, puedo empujar algunos de los bordes de la retina hacia mi campo visual.

POST-MYDRIATIC GLASSES
ANTEOJOS POSTMIDRIASIS

The eyes will be sensitive to light because of the medicine.
Los ojos van a estar sensibles a la luz debido a la medicina.

These sunglasses will help you outside. The medicine will last about three hours *(insert correct number)*.
Esos lentes de sol le ayudarán afuera. La medicina va a durar por tres horas.

Chapter 18
Special Ophthalmic Procedures

Capítulo 18
Procedimientos Oftálmicos Especiales

EPILATION
DEPILACIÓN

Some eyelashes are turned inward.
Algunas pestañas están volteadas hacia adentro.

They are bothering you, so I will remove them.
Ellas le están molestando, y por eso, voy a removerlas.

You may feel a tug for a second.
Usted puede sentir un tirón por un segundo.

Eyelashes typically grow back in 6-8 weeks. Hopefully it won't grow back curled against your eye surface. But if the lash seems to bother you again, please call the office.
Las pestañas por lo general crecen de nuevo en 6-8 semanas. Con suerte no crecerán de nuevo volteadas contra la superficie del ojo. Pero si las pestañas le vuelven a molestar, por favor llame a la oficina.

SUPERFICIAL FOREIGN BODY REMOVAL
EXTRACCIÓN SUPERFICIAL DE MATERIA EXTRAÑA

There is a small piece of something stuck to the outside part of the eye.
Hay un pedacito de algo pegado en la parte exterior del ojo.

I will remove it after giving you anesthetic drops.
Lo voy a quitar después de darle gotas anestésicas.

With the anesthetic, your eye should feel comfortable and allow me to quickly remove the foreign particle.
Con el anestésico, sus ojos deben sentirse cómodos y me permitirá remover la partícula extraña rápidamente.

Please hold your eye very still.
Por favor manténga su ojo quieto.

BANDAGE SOFT CONTACT LENS
LENTES DE CONTACTO DE VENDAJE

I am putting a contact lens over the eye like a bandage to help the healing.
Estoy poniendo un lente de contacto sobre el ojo como venda para ayudar la curación.

It will also make the eye feel better.
También mejorará la sensación del ojo.

When you return tomorrow, I may remove it or replace it.
Cuando vuelva mañana, puedo quitarlo o substituirlo.

If the lens falls out, call me—do not put it back in.
Si el lente se cae, llámeme—no se lo ponga de nuevo.

You will sleep with the lens.
Usted dormirá con el lente.

SCHIRMER TEAR TEST
PRUEBA SCHIRMER DE LÁGRIMAS

This piece of paper is for measuring the amount of tears you produce in five minutes.
Este pedazo de papel se utiliza para medir la cantidad de lágrimas que se producen en cinco minutos.

It may feel strange but it won't hurt you.
Se puede sentir extraño pero no le hará daño.

I will return in five minutes to remove the absorbent paper. Just look downward and refrain from moving your eyes around.
Regresaré en cinco minutos para quitar el papel absorbente. Sólo mire hacia abajo y evite que sus ojos se muevan.

Your eyes seem to produce a normal amount of tears.
Sus ojos parecen producir una cantidad normal de lágrimas.

Your eyes do not produce as much tears as I would expect.
Sus ojos no producen tantas lágrimas como yo hubiese esperado.

PUNCTAL OCCLUSION FOR KERATOCONJUNCTIVITIS SICCA
OCLUSIÓN PUNTAL PARA QUERATOCONJUTIVITIS SICCA

For dry eyes, I recommend a simple procedure to cover the part where tears leave the eye—the tear duct.
Para los ojos secos, le recomiendo un tratamiento sencillo para tapar la parte por donde las lágrimas salen del ojo—el lagrimal.

In this manner, the eyes will retain more tears for lubrication because they stay on the eye longer.
De esta manera, los ojos van a retener más lágrimas para lubricación porque se quedan más tiempo en el ojo.

The procedure helps the majority of patients.
El procedimiento ayuda a la mayoría de los pacientes.

I will place a plug in the tear duct.
Le voy a poner un tapón en el lagrimal.

PUNCTAL DILATION AND IRRIGATION
DILATACIÓN PUNTAL E IRRIGACIÓN

Everybody has a duct that connects the corner of the eye to the nose so that tears leave the eye to the nose.
Todas las personas tienen un conducto que conecta la esquina del ojo con la nariz para que las lágrimas salgan del ojo hasta la nariz.

In your case, this duct is blocked so the tears can't leave and the eye waters.
En su caso, este conducto está tapado y las lágrimas no pueden salir y el ojo llora.

I will (open/unblock) this duct with an instrument.
Voy a (abrir/destapar) el conducto con un instrumento.

Do you feel liquid in your mouth? Swallow it.
¿Siente líquido en la boca? Tráguelo.

OCULAR SURFACE IRRIGATION
IRRIGACIÓN DE LA SUPERFICIE OCULAR

I'm going to wash your eyes with saline. It will feel cold.
Voy a lavar sus ojos con solución salina. Se sentirá frío.

Please hold these tissues against your face to absorb the excess saline.
Por favor aguante estos pañitos contra su cara para absorber el exceso de la solución salina.

PRESSURE PATCHING
PARCHES DE PRESIÓN

I am applying a patch over the eye to help it heal.
Estoy aplicando un parche sobre el ojo para ayudarle a sanar.

The bandage should be a bit tight to help the eye.
La venda tiene que estar un poco apretada para ayudar al ojo.

When you return tomorrow, I will remove it.
Cuando usted regrese mañana, voy a removerla.

I will remove it when you come tomorrow.
Se la quitaré cuando venga mañana.

Meanwhile, for safety, avoid driving and working with heavy machinery.
Mientras tanto, por seguridad, evite conducir y trabajar con maquinaria pesada.

SUTURE BARB REMOVAL
EXTRACCIÓN DE PUNTADAS DE SUTURAS

You have sutures that are sticking out, and I am going to remove them.
Usted tiene suturas que están saliéndose, y voy a removerlas.

I will anesthetize the eye using eye drops.
Voy a anestesiar el ojo usando gotas.

You will need to use these antibiotic drops four times a day in the right eye.
Tendrá que usar estas gotas antibióticas cuatro veces al día en el ojo derecho.

FUNDUS PHOTOGRAPHY
FOTOGRAFÍA DEL FUNDUS

Photographs of the eye are medically necessary for documenting your condition.
Las fotografías del ojo son médicamente necesarias para documentar su condición.

Without the photographs, I cannot tell in the future if the condition is improving or worsening.
Sin las fotografías, no puedo saber en el futuro si la condición está mejorando o empeorando.

The information is necessary for determining the most appropriate treatment.
La información es necesaria para determinar el tratamiento más apropiado.

Chapter 19
Ophthalmic Dispensary

Capítulo 19
Dispensario Oftálmico

GENERAL
GENERAL

Take this prescription to the optician.
Lleve esta receta al óptico.

This is an expired prescription.
Esta es una receta vencida.

This prescription is expired.
Esta receta está vencida.

You need to have an exam to get a new prescription.
Usted tiene que hacerse un examen para obtener una
receta nueva.

**Take a seat here and in a moment, someone will be
with you (m./f.).**
Tome asiento aquí y en un momento, alguien (lo/la) van a
atender.

VISION PLAN COVERAGE
CUBIERTA DE PLAN DE VISIÓN

**Your insurance (*formal*/*informal*) does not include
benefits for frames and lenses.**
Su (aseguranza/seguro) no incluye beneficios para aros
y lentes.

Your eyes don't accept prescription lenses.
Sus ojos no aceptan lentes recetados.

There is no insurance that covers nonprescription sunglasses.
No hay ningún seguro que cubra los lentes de sol sin receta.

There is no insurance that covers nonprescription glasses.
No hay ningún seguro que cubra los anteojos sin recetas.

Sometimes patients with eyes like yours ask me if I can prescribe lenses. The answer is certainly "no."
A veces, los pacientes con ojos como los suyos me preguntan si les puedo recetar lentes. La respuesta es claramente "no".

Insurance companies and the laws don't permit this.
Las compañías de seguros y las leyes no permiten esto.

Still, I recommend that you buy nonprescription sunglasses because it is very important to protect your eyes from ultraviolet rays.
De todos modos, le recomiendo que compre los lentes de sol porque es muy importante proteger los ojos contra los rayos ultravioletas.

You can buy them nonprescription in any place.
Usted puede comprarlos sin receta en cualquier lugar.

Your insurance covers the exam, ordinary lenses, and frames.
Su seguro cubre el examen, los lentes comunes y aros.

The power of the lens is not covered by the insurance.
El aumento del lente no está cubierto por el seguro.

You have one hundred dollars credit for frames, renewable every two years.
Usted tiene un crédito de cien dólares para aros, renovable cada dos años.

You need to pay the deductible for the exam and for the materials.
Usted necesita pagar el deducible para el examen y para los materiales.

Premium lenses and frames cost more.
Los lentes y aros superiores cuestan más.

SELECTING FRAMES AND LENSES
SELECCIONAR LOS AROS Y LOS LENTES

To save you time, I am going to select five frames from our extensive selection which, based on my experience, will look the best on you.
Para ahorrarle tiempo, voy a escoger cinco aros de nuestra selección extensa, que basado en mi experiencia, se verán mejor en usted.

On your face, the best frame for you will have a round/oval/square shape.
En su cara, el mejor aro para usted tendrá una forma redonda/ovalada/cuadrada.

Those frames are too big/too small for you.
Esos aros son muy grandes/pequeños para usted.

Those frames do not allow enough viewing area with a bifocal or progressive lens.
Esos aros no permiten suficiente área de vista con un lente bifocal o progresivo.

The metal frames have adjustable nose pads.
Los aros de metal tienen patas en la parte de la nariz que se pueden ajustar.

Try these on. These frames look good on you.
Pruébese estos. Le quedan bien esos aros.

These rimless frames are more delicate, but they are very lightweight and stylish. You need special lenses with rimless frames so that the temples, which attach directly onto the lens, will not crack them.
Estos aros sin borde son más delicados, pero son muy livianos y elegantes. Usted necesitará lentes especiales con los aros sin bordes de manera que las patillas, que están conectadas al lente, no los agrieten.

These frames are made out of titanium, the strongest and lightest metal. It is also hypoallergenic, meaning that you will not develop any skin irritation wearing it.

Estos aros están hechos de titanio, el metal más fuerte y más liviano. También es hipoalergénico, lo que significa que usted no desarrollará una irritación en la piel usándolos.

These frames are more expensive, but they're worth it because they're of superior quality.

Esos aros son más caros, pero valen la pena porque la calidad es superior.

***Staff*: The doctor has prescribed a pair of distance glasses with a thin and light lens with an antireflective coating to make them as comfortable as possible. The cost of the pair of lenses comes to $215. Let us now move to the fun part of finding a frame!**

El doctor ha recetado un par de lentes de distancia con un lente fino y liviano con una capa antireflectiva para hacerlos tan cómodos como sea posible. El costo del par de lentes es de $215. ¡Vayamos ahora a la parte divertida de seleccionar un aro!

***Patient*: $215 seems too much. Is there anything less expensive?**

$215 parece ser demasiado. ¿Hay algo más barato?

***Staff*: I recommend staying with the lenses prescribed by the doctor. However if cost is a concern, you can have the thin and light lenses without the antireflective coating for $145. The antireflective treatment is beneficial because it makes the lenses look very clear while reducing reflections introduced by the lenses.**

Yo recomiendo que se quede con los lentes recetados por el doctor. Sin embargo, si el costo es una preocupación, usted puede tener los lentes finos y livianos sin la capa antireflectiva por $145. El tratamiento antireflectivo es beneficioso porque hace que los lentes se vean más claros mientras que reduce los reflejos introducidos por los lentes.

You need to leave the frames with us.
Usted tiene que dejar los aros con nosotros.

Because you are so heavily dependent on glasses, you really need to have a back-up pair.
Porque usted depende tanto de los anteojos, usted necesita tener un par de reemplazo.

Thinner lenses and an (antiscratch/antireflective) coating are options.
Los lentes más delgados y la capa (antirayazos/antireflectiva) son opciones.

The doctor has prescribed you high index lenses, which are thinner and lighter due to your strong prescription.
El doctor le ha recetado lentes de índice alto, los cuales son más finos y livianos debido a su receta tan fuerte.

High index lenses bend light more effectively than standard lenses. As a result, the lenses are thinner and usually light weight.
Los lentes de índice alto doblan la luz más efectivamente que los lentes estándares. Como resultado, los lentes son más finos y generalmente livianos.

I do not think you would be happy with the standard lenses because of their increased weight and thickness.
Yo no creo que usted estaría contento/a con los lentes estándares debido a su peso excesivo y su espesor.

This smaller frame will also reduce the edge thickness of your lenses.
Éste aro más pequeño también reducirá el espesor de sus lentes.

I recommend the antireflective coating because it makes the lenses almost invisible. It also reduces the reflections and ghost images normally introduced by the lenses.
Yo recomiendo la capa antireflectiva porque hace a los lentes casi invisibles. Ésta también reduce los reflejos y las imágenes fantasmas que normalmente son introducidas por los lentes.

Polycarbonate lenses are the standard lens for children because it is the safest, most shatter-resistant lens available. These lenses are also desirable because they are very light, they automatically come with a scratch-resistant coating, and full ultraviolet light protection.

Los lentes de policarbonato son los lentes estándares para los niños porque es el lente más seguro y más resistente a quebrantarse. Estos lentes también son deseables porque son muy livianos, automáticamente vienen con una capa antirayasos y protección ultravioleta completa.

Do you prefer (lenses that change color/ photochromatic lenses)?

¿Prefiere lentes (que cambian de color/fotocromáticos)?

The Transitions lenses are clear indoors and darken when exposed to sunlight. These lenses are excellent. Unlike previous generations of these lenses, they darken and lighten better and faster. However, they do not darken well inside of a car since your car windows will absorb most of the light that cause the lenses to change.

Los lentes Transitions son transparentes bajo techo y se oscurecen al estar expuestos a la luz solar. Estos lentes son excelentes. Contrario a las generaciones anteriores de estos lentes, éstos se oscurecen y se aclaran mejor y más rápido. Sin embargo, éstos no se oscurecen bien dentro de los autos porque las ventanas del auto absorberán la mayoría de la luz que causa que los lentes cambien.

Due to your high farsighted prescription, you need aspheric lenses. Aspheric lenses are special because the lenses are much thinner and lighter than standard lenses. They also reduce the distortion and unintended magnification effect while still bringing things into proper focus.

Debido a su receta hipermétrope, usted necesita lentes asféricos. Los lentes asféricos son especiales porque los lentes son más finos y livianos que los lentes estándares. Éstos también reducen la distorsión y el efecto de magnificación no intencional a la vez que permite enfocar correctamente en las cosas.

I want you to find a pair of glasses that you really like. If you don't, you won't want to use them even though you really need them!
Quiero que encuentre un par de anteojos que de verdad le gusten. ¡Si no, no va querer usarlos aunque de verdad los necesite!

Those glasses make you look like a movie star!
¡Esos anteojos la/lo hacen ver como una estrella de cine!

I am sure your friends will all like your stylish glasses!
¡Estoy seguro que a sus amigos les gustarán sus anteojos elegantes!

Glass lenses weigh twice as much as plastic lenses.
Los lentes de vidrio pesan dos veces más que los lentes de plástico.

They are also more prone to shattering.
También son más propensos a quebrarse.

Polarized sunglasses are the best. Unlike standard sunglasses, polarized lenses effectively reduce irritating glare reflecting from water, asphalt, and snow. You can tell that you have polarized lenses because any time you look at a cell phone display or liquid crystal watch display with them on, the screen will blacken when you rotate your head. With polarized lenses, you can also see optical defects in auto window glass. After trying polarized sunglasses, you won't go back to the standard sunglasses.
Los lentes de sol polarizados son los mejores. Contrario a los lentes de sol estándares, los lentes polarizados reducen efectivamente el resplandor irritante del agua, el asfalto y la nieve. Usted puede saber si tiene lentes polarizados porque cuando mira el despliegue de su teléfono celular o un reloj de cristal líquido con ellos, la pantalla se oscurecerá cuando gira su cabeza. Con los lentes polarizados, usted también puede ver defectos ópticos en el vidrio del auto. Después de probar los lentes de sol polarizados, usted no regresará a los lentes de sol estándares.

Progressive glasses are different from bifocals because there is no line running through the lens. They are the most advanced lens technology because they allow you to see clearly at all distances—far, intermediate, and up close—by moving the eyes to look through the appropriate part of the lens. Progressives work very well, but in the beginning it is common for new wearers to feel a bit nauseated, especially going up and down steps. That sensation goes away with continued wear.

Los lentes progresivos son diferentes de los bifocales porque no tienen una línea que cruza el lente. Estos son la tecnología más avanzada porque le permiten ver claramente a todas las distancias—lejos, intermedio y de cerca—moviendo sus ojos para ver a través de la parte apropiada del lente. Los lentes progresivos funcionan muy bien, pero al principio es común para los usuarios nuevos sentirse un poco nauseabundos, especialmente al subir y bajar escaleras. La sensación desaparece con el uso continuo.

The doctor has prescribed prism in your glasses. Prism does not bring things into focus, but it shifts what you see either left, right, up, or down, depending on what the doctor has prescribed. The image is shifted in the direction your eyes normally posture, in order to make it more comfortable for you to see.

El doctor ha recetado un prisma en sus anteojos. El prisma no ayuda a enfocar las cosas, pero mueve lo que usted ve hacia la izquierda, la derecha, arriba o abajo, dependiendo de qué el doctor recetó. La imagen se mueve en la dirección que sus ojos normalmente se dirigen, para poder hacerlo más cómodo para que usted vea.

The prism is necessary in your prescription. The cost of the prism is $20.

El prisma es necesario en su receta. El costo del prisma es de $20.

DISPENSING NEW GLASSES AND EXPLAINING ADAPTATION
DISPENSAR ANTEOJOS NUEVOS Y EXPLICAR LA ADAPTACIÓN

Use them (all the time/everyday) for one week so that you get used to them.
Úselos (siempre/todos los días) por una semana para acostumbrarse a ellos.

In the beginning, things may look a bit strange and distorted.
Al principio, es posible que las cosas se vean extrañas y distorsionadas.

But after one week with them, you should adapt and do well.
Pero después de una semana con ellos, debería adaptarse y andar bien.

It will take you longer to adjust to the new glasses if you keep taking them on and off. It will also take longer if you switch between using the new and old glasses.
Le va a tomar más tiempo adaptarse a los anteojos nuevos si usted continúa poniéndoselos y quitándoselos. También le va a tomar más tiempo si cambia entre los anteojos nuevos y los viejos.

In the unforeseen circumstance that you can't (adjust to/get acquainted with) them and you still feel bad after two weeks, return.
En caso que usted no pueda (acostumbrarse/imponerse) a ellos y todavía se siente mal después de dos semanas, regrese.

If you have diligently worn your new glasses for over one week and cannot comfortably wear them, please let us know. There are a very small number of patients that just cannot adjust to wearing progressive lenses. These special lenses are guaranteed, meaning that if you return them to us

within 60 days, we can change them for free into bifocal or standard single focus glasses.

Si usted ha usado diligentemente sus nuevos anteojos por más de una semana y no puede usarlos cómodamente, por favor déjenos saber. Hay un pequeño número de pacientes que simplemente no pueden ajustarse al usar los lentes progresivos. Estos lentes especiales están garantizados, lo que significa que si los devuelve dentro de 60 días, podemos cambiarlos de gratis a lentes bifocales o a lentes de visión sencilla.

The lenses were not made correctly.

Los lentes nunca fueron hechos correctamente.

Don't clean the lenses when they're dry. You need to clean them when they're wet.

No limpie los lentes cuando están secos. Hay que limpiarlos cuando están mojados.

Use liquid soap and water to clean your lenses. Make sure the soap is free of any creams or lotions, which may smear the lenses with oil.

Use jabón líquido y agua para limpiar sus lentes. Asegúrese que el jabón es libre de cremas o lociones, las cuales pueden manchar los lentes con aceite.

Due to the large difference between the prescriptions of your right and left lens, it usually is more difficult to adjust to your glasses. With a large asymmetry, each eye will see objects a different size and it may take time for the brain to learn to put the images together. Additionally, when you look off-center, one eye may see the object higher than the other eye.

Debido a las grandes diferencias entre las recetas en su lente derecho e izquierdo, generalmente es más difícil ajustarse a sus anteojos. Con una asimetría grande, cada ojo verá los objetos de tamaños diferentes y puede tomarle algún tiempo al cerebro aprender a unir las imágenes. Adicionalmente, cuando mira fuera de centro, un ojo puede ver un objeto más alto que el otro ojo.

You need slab-off prism in your glasses. This treatment adds a line which runs across the entire left/right lens. Without the slab-off prism, you may see double while reading. The slab-off prism vertically aligns each image so that your brain can put them together. The doubling effect is a result of your unique prescription where there is a huge asymmetry between the right and left lenses.

Usted necesita un prisma compensador en sus anteojos. Este tratamiento añade una línea que cruza el lente izquierdo/derecho completo. Sin el prisma compensador, usted podría ver doble cuando lee. El prisma compensador alinea cada imagen verticalmente de manera que su cerebro pueda unirlas. El efecto de visión doble es el resultado de una receta única donde hay una asimetría enorme entre el lente derecho y el izquierdo.

Chapter 20
Working with Children

Capítulo 20
Trabajando con Niños

BUILDING RAPPORT
DESARROLLANDO UNA BUENA RELACIÓN

How's it going, my little one (m./f.)?
¿Cómo andas, mi amigo/a?

What are your favorite things to do in school?
¿Cuáles son tus cosas favoritas para hacer en la escuela?

What hobbies or sports do you enjoy?
¿Qué pasatiempos o deportes disfrutas?

Do you have any brothers or sisters?
¿Tienes hermanos o hermanas?

How old are you?
¿Cuántos años tienes?

Give me a smile.
Dame una sonrisa.

Why are you so afraid?
¿Por qué tienes tanto miedo?

If you're good, I'll give you a sticker.
Si te portas bien, te voy a dar una calcomanía.

What do you want to be when you grow up?
¿Qué quieres ser cuando seas grande?

Have you gone to the movies?
¿Has ido al cine?

With this instrument, I can see all of your thoughts. Do you believe it?
Con este instrumento, puedo ver todos tus pensamientos. ¿Lo puedes creer?

Are you embarrassed?
¿Estás avergonzado?

Do you cause trouble at home?
¿Haces travesuras en la casa?

Do you like jokes?
¿Te gustan (los chistes/las bromas)?

Why are you smiling?
¿Por qué estás sonriendo?

GENERAL
GENERAL

Directed to parent: **Have your child (m./f.) sit in your lap.**
Siente a su niño/a en sus piernas.

Directed to parent: **Does your child's (m./f.) eye wander? Inward (cross-eyed) or outward (wall-eyed)?**
¿Se le bizca un ojo a su hijo/a? ¿Hacia adentro o hacia fuera?

To make you taller on the exam chair, I'd like you to sit on your knees.
Para hacerte más alto/a en la silla de examen, quisiera que te sentaras sobre tus rodillas.

Can you sit cross-legged?
¿Puedes sentarte con las piernas cruzadas?

Do not touch the instruments, because if you break it you'll have to pay for it!
No toques los instrumentos, porque si los rompes, ¡vas a tener que pagarlos!

Good job!
¡Buen trabajo!

Sit still. Come with me.
Siéntate quieto. Ven conmigo.

Give me your hand.
Dame tu mano.

Don't do that, my little one (m./f.).
No hagas eso, mi amigo/a.

Don't rub (your eyes).
No te talles/frotes (tus ojos).

Tell me these letters. Do the best you can.
Dime estas letras. Haz lo mejor que puedas.

It won't hurt you at all.
No te va a doler nada.

Pay attention. Listen to me (*harsh*)!
Pon atención. ¡Hazme caso!

Don't look at my light. Look for the red and green.
No mires mi luz. Mira el rojo y verde.

OCCLUSION THERAPY FOR AMBLYOPIA
TERAPIA DE OCLUSIÓN PARA LA AMBLIOPÍA

Directed to parent: **Your daughter/son needs to use a patch on her/his right/left eye to strengthen her/his left/right eye.**
Su hija/o necesita usar un parche sobre su ojo derecho/izquierdo para fortalecer su ojo izquierdo/derecho.

The left/right eye hasn't been working.
El ojo izquierdo/derecho no ha estado trabajando.

The result is that the vision in this eye has not developed normally.
El resultado es que la vista en este ojo no se ha desarrollado normalmente.

The patch will force the weak eye to work.
El parche va a forzar al ojo débil a trabajar.

You need to put the patch over the eye every third day, full-time during the day.
Debe poner el parche sobre el ojo cada tercer día, todo el tiempo durante el día.

It is important to start this treatment immediately and follow the regimen carefully until the next visit.
Es importante empezar este tratamiento inmediatamente y seguir el régimen con cuidado hasta la próxima visita.

GENERAL
GENERAL

The main reason you have… is because…
La razón principal que tiene … es porque …

Everything inside the eye is healthy—the retina, the blood vessels, and the optic nerves.
Todo dentro del ojo está sano—la retina, los vasos sanguíneos y los nervios ópticos.

Even though your eyes are healthy, they are not well focused. That's why glasses are necessary to clear things up.
Aunque sus ojos están sanos, no están bien enfocados. Por eso se necesitan anteojos para aclarar las cosas.

The condition of your eyes is stable.
La condición de sus ojos está estable.

Don't worry.
No se preocupe.

Your condition is in an advanced state.
Su condición está en un estado avanzado.

Fortunately, you don't have any eye disease.
Afortunadamente, no tiene ninguna enfermedad en los ojos.

I'm sorry but the eye is damaged.
Lo siento pero el ojo está dañado.

Unfortunately, there is no treatment to repair your vision.
Desafortunadamente, no hay tratamiento para reparar su visión.

The only treatment is to protect the other eye.
El único tratamiento es proteger el otro ojo.

It is not worthwhile to do surgery now.
No vale la pena hacer la cirugía ahora.

WHEN SURGERY IS INDICATED
CUANDO SE RECOMIENDA CIRUGÍA

You would benefit greatly from eye surgery to treat this problem.
Usted podría beneficiarse grandemente de la cirugía ocular para tratar este problema.

As with any surgery, there are some inherent risks, including the possibility of infection and an outcome that is not optimal. However, at this point, I believe the benefits greatly outweigh the risks. I would recommend the surgery to any friend or family member in the same situation.
Como con cualquier cirugía, hay algunos riesgos inherentes, incluyendo la posibilidad de infección y un resultado que no es óptimo. Sin embargo, en este punto, yo creo que los beneficios superan a los riesgos. Yo recomendaría esta cirugía a cualquier amigo o familiar en la misma situación.

The surgery itself does not take long and causes minimal discomfort because your eye is anesthetized during the procedure. You will go home the same day.
La cirugía misma no toma mucho tiempo y causa molestia mínima porque su ojo está anestesiado durante el procedimiento. Usted regresará a casa el mismo día.

You are not allowed to rub your eye vigorously afterwards. Avoid heavy lifting, stooping, or bending over for one week following surgery.
No se le permite frotar su ojo vigorosamente después de la cirugía. Evite levantar cosas pesadas, encorvarse o doblarse por una semana después de la cirugía.

You will need to have a driver bring you to and from the surgery.
Usted necesitará que un chofer lo traiga y regrese de la cirugía.

I will prescribe medicines for you to use after your surgery.
Voy a recetarle medicinas para que las use después de la cirugía.

I will have one of my staff explain to you the informed consent form, which goes over the indications, risks, benefits, and alternatives to having eye surgery.
Voy a hacer que alguien de mi equipo le explique el formulario de consentimiento informado, el cual cubre las indicaciones, los riesgos, los beneficios y las alternativas de tener cirugía ocular.

POSTOPERATIVE CARE
CUIDADO POSTOPERATORIO

Everything appears fine, but you need to wait for it to get better.
Todo parece estar bien, pero tiene que esperar para que se le mejore.

The wound is (not) healing as (I/one) would have expected.
La lesión (no) está mejorando como (yo/se) esperaba.

Have patience. Your vision will improve little by little.
Tenga paciencia. Su visión mejorará poco a poco.

You need to avoid swimming and direct water contact with the eye until the next visit.
Usted debería evitar el nadar y el contacto directo con agua en el ojo hasta la próxima visita.

MEDICATION
MEDICAMENTOS

Use these drops four times a day in both eyes until you finish the bottle.
Use estas gotas cuatro veces al día en los dos ojos hasta que termine la botella.

Shake the drops before applying to the eye.
Agite las gotas antes de aplicarlas al ojo.

Shake well and keep refrigerated.
Agite bien y manténgalas refrigeradas.

This prescription can be refilled two times.
Esta medicina puede surtirse dos veces.

Don't stop taking this medication suddenly.
No deje de usar esta medicina repentinamente.

Don't use it more than four times a day until the next visit.
No la use más de cuatro veces al día hasta la próxima visita.

These drops are for stopping the inflammation of the eyes.
Estas gotas son para parar la inflamación de los ojos.

Remember to shake the bottle before using.
Recuerde agitar la botella antes de usar la medicina.

When you finish them according to the instructions, don't use them again without my direction.
Cuando las termine según las instrucciones, no las use más sin mi indicación.

This medication is for relieving your pain.
Esta medicina es para aliviarle el dolor.

Put a bit of this ointment on the edge of your eyelids at night.
Ponga un poco de esta pomada sobre la orilla de sus párpados por la noche.

Take one pill four times a day.
Tome una pastilla cuatro veces al día.

Take at mealtime.
Tómese a la hora de las comidas.

Use the medication as directed.
Use el medicamento según se le indicó.

ARTIFICIAL TEARS
LÁGRIMAS ARTIFICIALES

I recommend that you use artificial tears to reduce the irritation and dryness.
Le recomiendo que use las lágrimas artificiales para disminuir la irritación y resequedad.

These drops are for lubrication and to wash the eyes.
Estas gotas son para la lubricación y para lavar los ojos.

They will not stop the redness completely because they contain no medicine.
No quitarán el enrojecimiento del todo porque no hay medicina en los ingredientes.

They are very natural.
Son muy naturales.

One brand of artificial tears is called Refresh Tears.
Una marca de lágrimas artificiales se llama Refresh Tears.

This brand is unique because it does not contain any preservative, and therefore, it's possible to use it as frequently as you like.
Esta marca es única porque no contiene ningún preservativo, y por eso, es posible usarla tan frecuentemente como guste.

You can buy them in any pharmacy without a prescription.
Puede comprarlas en cualquier farmacia sin receta.

SUN PROTECTION
PROTECCIÓN SOLAR

It is important to protect your eyes from ultraviolet rays.
Es importante proteger sus ojos contra los rayos ultravioletas.

With too much exposure to ultraviolet rays, the skin can burn.
Al exponerse demasiado a los rayos ultravioletas, la piel se puede quemar.

Ultraviolet rays damage the eyes just as they do the skin.
Los rayos ultravioletas causan daño a los ojos al igual que en la piel.

For example, there is a relation between these rays and tumors of the eyelids, pingueculae/ pterygia*; cataracts, and problems of the cornea and retina.
Por ejemplo, hay una relación entre estos rayos y los tumores de los párpados, las (pingüéculas/pterigiones/ carnosidades), las cataratas y los problemas de la córnea y la retina.

The eyes are very sensitive.
Los ojos son muy sensibles.

When you are outside, wear a hat and put on sunglasses.
Cuando esté afuera, use un sombrero y póngase los lentes de sol.

REFRACTIVE ERROR
ERROR REFRACTIVO

You have myopia, or nearsightedness. With this condition, close objects are seen well, but faraway objects are blurry.
Usted tiene miopía o visión corta. Con esta condición, los objetos próximos se ven bien, pero los objetos lejanos se ven borrosos.

---

* *Pingueculae* and *pterygia* are so common among Hispanics that most of them know the equivalent word, *carnosidad.*

You have farsightedness. With this condition, it is more comfortable to see faraway objects than up close. To keep things clear, you are exerting excessive force, which can cause discomfort.

Usted tiene hipermetropía. Con esta condición, es más cómodo ver los objetos lejanos que los próximos. Para mantener las cosas claras, usted está haciendo un esfuerzo excesivo, lo que puede causar incomodidad.

You have a condition called *astigmatism*. Normally, the front of the eye is a perfect sphere, like a baseball. But your cornea is a bit irregular in form, like a spoon. Consequently, the eye does not focus images clearly, and your vision is blurry.

Usted tiene una condición que se llama *astigmatismo*. Normalmente, el frente del ojo es una esfera perfecta, como una pelota de béisbol. Pero su córnea tiene una forma un poco irregular, como de cuchara. Por lo tanto, el ojo no enfoca las imágenes claramente, y su visión es borrosa.

It is a myth that glasses change the power the eyes need.

Es un mito que los anteojos cambian el aumento que necesitan los ojos.

If the eyes change power, they will do so with or without glasses.

Si los ojos cambian de aumento, lo harán con o sin anteojos.

Therefore, I recommend that you use glasses because they are more comfortable for the eyes.

Entonces, le recomiendo que use los anteojos porque son más cómodos para los ojos.

PRESBYOPIA
PRESBICIA

Like everyone, when you were a kid (m./f.), you were able to focus real close. But with time, this point of focus moves back, little by little.

Como todas las personas, cuando usted era niño/a podía enfocar muy de cerca. Pero con el tiempo ese punto de enfoque se mueve hacia atrás poco a poco.

This happens to everyone; there are no exceptions.
Esto les pasa a todos; no hay excepciones.

Close to the age of forty, this point is like this
  (*demonstrate at arm's length*).
Cerca de los cuarenta años de edad, ese punto está así.

The arms are not long enough to read clearly.
Los brazos no son suficientemente largos para leer
  claramente.

This is the time for (help/a little help) to see up
  (close/diminutive form of "close").
Ya es tiempo de una (ayuda/ayudita) para ver de
  (cerca/cerquita).

Now you need help to focus.
Ahora usted necesita ayuda para enfocar.

Now you need glasses for reading.
Ya necesita anteojos para leer.

Now there is an indication for reading glasses.
Ahora se pueden recomendar los anteojos para leer.

**The most common treatment for presbyopia is to use
bifocals. These lenses have two parts because now
your eyes require two different powers. The top part
is for seeing distance, and the bottom part is for
seeing close-up. It is convenient because one doesn't
have to always change between two different pairs of
glasses.**
El tratamiento más común para la presbicia es usar bifocales.
  Estos lentes tienen dos partes porque ahora sus ojos
  requieren dos aumentos diferentes. La parte de arriba es para
  ver de lejos, y la parte de abajo es para ver de cerca. Es
  conveniente porque no se necesita siempre estar cambiando
  entre dos pares de anteojos diferentes.

**The most modern lenses are the progressive lenses.
These are like bifocals without the line. With
progressives, when you look in front, you see well**

far away. When you are lowering the eyes you have
more and more power for focusing up close.

Los lentes más modernos son los lentes progresivos. Son como
bifocales pero sin la línea. Con los progresivos, al mirar
derecho se ve bien lo de lejos. Al bajar los ojos, hay más y
más aumento para ver de cerca.

Only parts of the lenses are useful, and for this reason,
it will take about one week of daily use to get (used
to/accustomed to) them.

Solamente algunas partes de los lentes son útiles, y por lo
tanto, tardará alrededor de una semana de uso diario para
(imponerse/acostumbrarse) a ellos.

Furthermore, because progressives are of superior
technology, they are more expensive than
bifocals.

Además, porque los progresivos son de tecnología superior, son
más caros que los bifocales.

CONTACT LENSES
LENTES DE CONTACTO

There are two general classes of contact
lenses: (rigid/hard) and (soft/soft). In your case,
I can prescribe either to correct your vision.
Most patients choose soft contact lenses because they
are more comfortable in the beginning. But rigid
lenses are equally comfortable after adapting to them
for a few weeks. There are benefits to rigid contact
lenses. For many patients, they are more durable,
healthier, and offer better vision than soft contact
lenses.

Hay dos clases generales de lentes de contacto: (rígidos/duros)
y (blandos/suaves). En su caso, puedo recetar cualquiera para
corregir la visión. La mayoría de los pacientes escogen lentes
de contacto blandos porque son más cómodos al principio.
Pero los lentes rígidos son igualmente cómodos después de
adaptarse por unas semanas. Hay beneficios con lentes de
contacto rígidos. Para muchos pacientes, ellos son más
duraderos, sanos, y ofrecen mejor visión que los lentes de
contacto blandos.

In your case, I recommend rigid gas-permeable contact lenses because I think they will offer you the best vision and eye health.

En su caso, le recomiendo los lentes de contacto rígidos de gas permeable porque creo que le ofrecerán la mejor visión y salud ocular.

If the eye gets red or you feel discomfort while using the lenses, remove them immediately.

Si el ojo se enrojece o siente molestia mientras usa los lentes, quíteselos inmediatamente.

If the problem continues once the lenses are out, call me at once.

Si el problema continúa aún quitados los lentes, llámeme de inmediato.

Always wash your hands before touching the lenses. Use soap that is free of lotion and fragrance.

Siempre lave sus manos antes de tocar los lentes. Use jabón libre de lociones y fragancias.

Put on your makeup after putting in the contact lenses.

Póngase el maquillaje después de ponerse los lentes de contacto.

There are now certain soft contact lenses approved for up to thirty days of continuous wear. These are lenses which you sleep with without removing. Even though these new lenses are extremely permeable to oxygen, they are not as safe as lenses removed on a daily basis. Waste products trapped underneath these lenses for extended periods of time cause eye irritation, even though the lenses transmit oxygen freely.

Ahora hay ciertos lentes de contactos blandos que están aprobados para hasta treinta días de uso continuo. Estos son lentes con los que duerme sin tener que quitárselos. Aunque estos nuevos lentes son extremadamente permeables al oxígeno, no son tan seguros como los lentes que se quitan diariamente. Los productos de desecho que se quedan atrapados debajo de estos lentes por periodos extensos de tiempo causan irritación del ojo, a pesar que los lentes transmiten oxígeno libremente.

Never use tap water, distilled water, or homemade saline solutions with your lenses.
Nunca use agua de la llave, agua destilada o soluciones salinas caseras con sus lentes.

Your soft contact lenses require daily removal for cleaning and disinfection.
Sus lentes de contacto blandos requieren que se los quite diariamente para su limpieza y desinfección.

With the lenses in the palm of a hand, apply the cleaning solution, rubbing it against the lens for twenty seconds. Take care not to scratch or break them with the fingernails.
Con los lentes en la palma de una mano, aplique la solución limpiadora, frotándola contra el lente por veinte segundos. Tenga cuidado de no rayarlos o romperlos con las uñas.

After cleaning them, rinse them with a commercial saline solution and then disinfect them.
Después de limpiarlos, enjuáguelos con una solución salina comercial y luego desinféctelos.

Each day, clean and air-dry the lens case. Replace it periodically.
Diariamente, limpie y seque al aire el estuche de sus lentes. Reemplácelo periódicamente.

You need to replace the lenses every (two weeks/months/three months).
Usted necesita reemplazar los lentes cada (dos semanas/mes/ tres meses).

When lenses are worn for a longer duration than recommended, there is a greater risk of redness, irritation, and infection.
Cuando los lentes se usan por más tiempo que el recomendado, hay un mayor riesgo de enrojecimiento, irritación e infección.

You would make an excellent candidate for contact lens wear. Unlike glasses, contacts would offer you improved peripheral vision, helping with sports and outdoor activities.

Usted sería un candidato excelente para los lentes de contacto. Contrario a los anteojos, los lentes de contacto le ofrecerán mejor visión periférica, le ayudarán con los deportes y las actividades recreativas.

In order to move forward with contact lens wear, you need to undergo contact lens prescribing. You have already had an eye examination. Based on my exam findings, you would do best wearing (soft disposable contact lenses/rigid gas-permeable contacts). Unlike with glasses, contact lens prescribing is different because it is a process that takes longer. To begin, I will need to apply a diagnostic contact lenses on your eye. These initial lenses may not necessarily sit properly on the eye, nor give optimal vision. However, they allow me to determine what you may need for optimal comfort and vision. Most importantly, I must make sure the lenses are healthy for you to wear in order to minimize the risk of unnecessary redness, irritation, and infection. One of my staff will teach how to properly apply, remove, and care for your contact lenses. Learning is fun yet sometimes frustrating. But you will probably pick up the technique fairly quickly. After receiving instructions on contact lens care and a wearing schedule, you will need to return for a progress visit in about one week. Please come in wearing your contact lenses at that time.

Para poder continuar con el uso de lentes de contacto, usted necesita recibir una receta de lentes de contacto. Usted ya tuvo su examen de la vista. Basado en los hallazgos de mi examen, usted estaría mejor usando lentes de contacto (blandos desechables/rígidos de gas permeable). Contrario a los anteojos, las recetas para los lentes de contacto son diferentes porque el proceso toma más tiempo. Para comenzar, voy a tener que poner un lente de contacto de diagnóstico en su ojo. Estos lentes iniciales puede que no necesariamente encajen bien en el ojo o provean la mejor visión. Sin embargo, me permiten determinar qué usted

puede necesitar para la comodidad y visión óptima.
Más importantemente, tengo que asegurarme que los
lentes son saludables para que usted los use para minimizar
el riesgo de enrojecimiento, irritación e infección innecesaria.
Alguien de mi equipo le enseñará cómo aplicar, remover
y cuidar correctamente sus lentes de contacto. Aprender
puede ser divertido pero frustrante a veces. Pero usted
probablemente aprenderá la técnica rápidamente. Después
de recibir las instrucciones para el cuidado de los lentes
de contacto y el horario de uso, usted tendrá que regresar
para una visita de progreso en aproximadamente una
semana. Por favor venga usando sus lentes de
contacto.

**If you experience unusual redness, pain, discharge,
decreased vision, or light sensitivity, please remove
your lenses immediately. If the symptoms persist
without improvement, please call the office.**
Si usted sufre de enrojecimiento, dolor, descarga, disminución
en su visión o sensibilidad a la luz inusual, por favor quítese
sus lentes inmediatamente. Si los síntomas persisten sin
mejoría, por favor llame a la oficina.

**The safest wear of contact lenses remains daily
removal. There are now contact lenses designed
and approved for continuous wear. These new lenses
are very oxygen transmissible. However, they still
suffer from an increased incidence of redness and
irritation, and possibly infection. When a lens is
on the eye for such an extended period of time,
waste products can accumulate underneath
the lens without getting flushed out, leading to eye
irritation.**
El uso más seguro de los lentes de contacto sigue siendo el
quitárselos diariamente. Ahora hay lentes de contacto
diseñados y aprobados para uso continuo. Estos lentes nuevos
transmiten mucho oxígeno. Sin embargo, todavía sufren de
una incidencia mayor de enrojecimiento e irritación, y
posiblemente infección. Cuando un lente está en el ojo por
un periodo extenso de tiempo, los productos de desecho se
pueden acumular debajo del lente sin ser eliminados,
produciendo irritación en el ojo.

REFRACTIVE SURGERY
CIRUGÍA REFRACTIVA

For many people, refractive surgery is a relatively safe, attractive, and effective method of visual correction.
Para muchas personas, la cirugía refractiva es un método relativamente seguro, atractivo, y eficiente para la corrección visual.

However, if you need guaranteed results, refractive surgery is not an appropriate option.
Sin embargo, si usted necesita resultados garantizados, la cirugía refractiva no es una opción apropiada.

It is important that you have sensible expectations.
Es importante que tenga expectaciones sensatas.

The goal of refractive surgery is not to throw away your contact lenses or glasses completely.
La meta de la cirugía refractiva no es deshacerse de los lentes de contacto o los anteojos por completo.

The true goal of refractive surgery is to reduce your dependency on contact lenses and glasses and improve your visual function.
La meta verdadera de la cirugía refractiva es reducir su dependencia de los lentes de contacto y mejorar su función visual.

With refractive surgery you will depend less on your glasses, but you may still sometimes need them.
Con la cirugía refractiva usted va a depender menos de sus anteojos, pero todavía es posible que los vaya a necesitar algunas veces.

It is not sensible that you will never need glasses again.
No es sensato que nunca vaya a necesitar sus anteojos.

This is a message different from the advertising.
Esto es un mensaje diferente de lo que dice la propaganda.

I expect the surgery to improve your natural vision.
Espero que la cirugía mejore su visión natural.

It is realistic to expect to drive, swim, and watch television without needing to use glasses or contacts.
Es realista esperar manejar, nadar y ver televisión sin necesidad de anteojos o lentes de contacto.

Although the laser and surgical technique are precise, there is some variability in the final outcome due to individual healing. Results differ from person to person. Even within the same person, usually one eye turns out better or worse than the other.
Aunque las técnicas de rayos láser y quirúrgicas son precisas, hay cierta variabilidad en el resultado final debido a la cicatrización individual. Los resultados difieren de persona a persona. Aún con la misma persona, generalmente un ojo sale mejor o peor que el otro.

To attain the best vision, you will still likely need some lenses.
Para alcanzar la visión óptima, probablemente usted todavía necesitará los anteojos.

It is possible that your vision will not be as good as when you use contacts or glasses.
Existe la posibilidad de que su visión no sea tan buena como cuando usa los lentes de contacto o anteojos.

Be very careful where you go. Generally, you should avoid places that use coupons and advertise low prices.
Tenga mucho cuidado a donde usted va. Generalmente, debería evitar los lugares que utilizan cupones y anuncian precios bajos.

I recommend Dr. Sandy T. Feldman. She is an excellent refractive surgeon. You can set up a complimentary consultation with her by calling her office.
Yo le recomiendo a la Dra. Sandy T. Feldman. Ella es una cirujana refractiva excelente. Usted puede establecer una consulta complementaria con ella llamando a su oficina.

Our office will share your existing exam information with Dr. Feldman so that you won't need every single eye measurement repeated.
Nuestra oficina compartirá la información existente de su examen con la Dra. Feldman para que usted no tenga que volver a obtener cada medida ocular.

You need to review the informed consent form, which more completely describes the risks, benefits, and alternatives to refractive surgery.
Usted necesita revisar el formulario de consentimiento informado, que describe más detalladamente los riesgos, beneficios y las alternativas de la cirugía refractiva.

I wish I could promise you that your vision would certainly come out perfectly. However, that would be unrealistic. It is my desire to fully inform you of the possible outcomes from surgery, including the potential risks. It is not reasonable to expect a problem. Yet it remains a real possibility.
Quisiera poder prometerle que su visión ciertamente quedará perfecta. Sin embargo, eso sería poco realista. Mi deseo es informarle de los posibles resultados de la cirugía, incluyendo los posibles riesgos. No es razonable esperar un problema, pero permanece una posibilidad real.

You can throw away a bad pair of glasses or contact lenses. But you can't throw away bad surgery.
Usted puede tirar unos anteojos o un par de lentes de contacto malos. Pero usted no puede tirar una mala cirugía.

Look for experience, quality, and service.
Busque la experiencia, la calidad y el servicio.

Would you like an information packet?
¿Quiere un paquete de información?

In the early recovery period, it is normal to experience light sensitivity, fluctuating vision, dryness symptoms, and night vision problems.
En el periodo de recuperación temprana, es normal que sufra sensibilidad a la luz, visión que fluctúa, síntomas de resequedad y problemas con su visión de noche.

I expect your vision to stay similar to where it is at today's visit, but since I can't fully predict how your eyes will respond to the treatment, I need to see you for a scheduled progress visit in three weeks.

Espero que su visión permanezca similar a como está en la visita de hoy, pero como yo no puedo predecir cómo sus ojos responderán al tratamiento, voy a tener que verlo en una visita programada dentro de tres semanas.

It is important for you to refrain from vigorously rubbing your eyes the first two weeks after surgery. The first week, you will have goggles to wear at nighttime to prevent you from inadvertently rubbing your eye while you sleep.

Es importante que evite frotar sus ojos vigorosamente las primeras dos semanas después de la cirugía. La primera semana, usted tendrá que usar gafas protectoras en las noches para evitar frotarse los ojos accidentalmente mientras duerme.

Chapter 22
Explanations for Specific Conditions

Capítulo 22
Explicaciones para Condiciones Específicas

BLEPHARITIS
BLEFARITIS

Everybody has oil glands in their eyelids.
Todos tenemos glándulas de aceite en los párpados.

Sometimes, what can happen is that the glands plug up or there is too much bacteria on the eyelids.
A veces, lo que puede suceder es que las glándulas se tapan o hay demasiada bacteria sobre los párpados.

This is the reason for your irritation.
Ésta es la razón de su irritación.

It is necessary to put towels with warm water over the eyelids two times each day, five minutes each time.
Es necesario poner toallas con agua tibia sobre los párpados dos veces cada día, cinco minutos cada vez.

Clean the edges of the eyelids near the eyelashes with OCuSOFT for one minute.
Limpie las orillas de los párpados cerca de las pestañas con OCuSOFT por un minuto.

Afterwards, rinse the closed eyes with warm water very well.
Después, enjuague los ojos cerrados con agua tibia muy bien.

Also, use artificial tears frequently.
También, use las lágrimas artificiales con frecuencia.

Follow this schedule for one month consistently.
Siga esta receta por un mes consistentemente.

If afterwards the symptoms persist, return and I will prescribe (drops/pills).
Si después de un tiempo todavía existen los síntomas, regrese y le recetaré unas (gotas/pastillas).

ALLERGIC CONJUNCTIVITIS
CONJUNTIVITIS ALÉRGICA

You have allergies in your eyes, and that is why your eyes itch.
Usted tiene alergias en sus ojos, y por eso la comezón en sus ojos.

I'm going to prescribe some drops, called Patanol, for diminishing the symptoms.
Voy a recetar unas gotas, llamadas Patanol, para disminuir los síntomas.

One uses these drops twice a day.
Se echan estas gotas dos veces al día.

In the morning, put a drop in each eye.
En la mañana, ponga una gota en cada ojo.

In the evening, put the drops in again.
Por la noche, otra vez, ponga las gotas.

Use the drops for at least one month.
Use las gotas por lo menos un mes.

Each day, the medicine will help you more and more.
Cada día, la medicina va a ayudarle más y más.

These drops are very good and are very safe.
Estas gotas son muy buenas y son muy seguras.

VASOCONSTRICTOR OVERUSE
ABUSO DE UN VASOCONSTRICTOR

Your eyes are red because you are using the Visine drops too much.

Sus ojos están rojos porque está usando las gotas Visine demasiado.

I recommend that you don't use them more than three times a day, or better, only once in a while.

Le recomiendo que no las use más de tres veces al día, o mejor, solamente de vez en cuando.

With time, the eyes adapt to the medicine, and you need to use more and more to achieve the same level of whiteness.

Con el tiempo, los ojos se adaptan a la medicina, y usted necesita usar más y más para lograr el mismo nivel de blancura.

With too much Visine, the eyes again become red when they adapt to the drops.

Con demasiado Visine, los ojos otra vez se ponen rojos cuando se adaptan a las gotas.

One needs to put less and less Visine each day, little by little.

Hay que poner menos y menos Visine cada día, poco a poco.

And in its place, start to put in artificial tears.

Y en su lugar, empiece a poner las lágrimas artificiales.

PINGUECULAE AND PTERYGIA*
PINGUÉCULAS Y PTERIGIONES
(CARNOSIDADES)

You have a (pinguecula/pterygium). This is very common, and most of the time, there are no consequences.

---

* *Pingueculae* and *pterygia* are so common among Hispanics that most of them know the equivalent word, *carnosidad.*

Usted tiene (una pinguécula/un pterigión/una carnosidad). Esto
   es muy común, y la mayoría de las veces, no hay
   consecuencias.

**The cause is irritation, like contamination in the air,
   dust in the air, and ultraviolet rays.**
La causa es irritación, como la contaminación en el aire, el
   polvo en el aire y los rayos ultravioletas.

**With too much irritation, the (pinguecula/pterygium)
   will grow.**
Con demasiada irritación, (la pinguécula/el pterigión/la
   carnosidad) va a crecer.

**If it grows enough, it can advance into the
   cornea, which is the clear part in front of
   the eye.**
Si le crece mucho, puede avanzar a la córnea, que es la parte
   transparente en el frente del ojo.

**In some of these cases, the pterygium grows
   into the center of vision, and hence affects
   the vision.**
En algunos de estos casos, (el pterigión/la carnosidad) crece
   hasta el centro de la vista, y entonces afecta la visión.

This is a problem.
Esto es un problema.

**If the pterygium is big enough, there is an indication
   for a simple surgery.**
Si (el pterigión/la carnosidad) es suficientemente grande,
   entonces se recomienda una cirugía sencilla.

**But for you right now, there is no indication for
   surgery.**
Pero por ahora, no hay indicación para cirugía.

**Just continue with the artificial tears and protect your
   eyes with sunglasses.**
Sólo continúe con las lágrimas artificiales y proteja sus ojos con
   lentes de sol.

You need to return in one year because I want to see if the (pinguecula/pterygium) is growing.
Usted debe regresar en un año porque quiero ver si (la pinguécula/el pterigión/la carnosidad) está creciendo.

Now is the time for surgery.
Ahora es cuando se debe operar.

It is big enough, and if you don't do anything, it will probably affect your vision.
Está suficientemente grande, y si no se hace nada, probablemente afectará su visión.

But this operation, like all surgeries, is no guarantee because in thirty percent of cases the pterygium returns within five years.
Pero esta operación, como todas las cirugías, no es una garantía porque en un treinta por ciento de los casos (el pterigión/la carnosidad) regresa dentro de cinco años.

And with surgery, there is the minimal risk for infection and bad outcomes.
Y con la cirugía, hay un riesgo mínimo de infección y resultados malos.

But those cases are rare.
Pero esos casos son raros.

Right now, the positives for surgery outweigh the negatives.
Ahora mismo, los positivos para la cirugía pesan más que los negativos.

Later, you need to make an appointment to consult with the surgeon.
Después, tiene que hacer una cita para consultar con el cirujano.

CATARACTS AND SURGERY
CATARATAS Y CIRUGÍA

You have the beginning of cataracts.
Usted tiene el comienzo de cataratas.

Right now they are not affecting your vision, but in the future it's possible (they will affect it).
Ahora no están afectando su visión, pero en el futuro es posible que sí (le afecten).

Cataracts are very common.
Las cataratas son muy comunes.

They exist when the crystalline lens (becomes cloudy/opacifies/has an opacity).
Existen cuando el lente cristalino (se nubla/se opaca/tiene opacidad).

Many older people have cataracts.
Muchas personas mayores tienen cataratas.

With age, the hair color changes.
Con la edad, el color del pelo cambia.

And with the crystalline lens, the same thing—it begins to get more yellow and more opaque with age.
Y con el lente cristalino, lo mismo—empieza a hacerse más amarillo y más opaco con la edad.

The cataracts aren't mature yet, but perhaps in five years they will be.
Las cataratas todavía no están maduras, pero tal vez en cinco años sí lo estarán.

They still aren't appropriate for operating.
Todavía no están apropiadas para operarse.

Just return each year for an eye checkup.
Solamente regrese cada año para una revisión de los ojos.

We are going to (observe them/be observing them) (*referring to the cataracts*).
Vamos a (observarlas/estarlas observando).

The operation for removing the crystalline lens is very easy nowadays.
La cirugía para quitar el lente cristalino es muy fácil hoy en día.

It's totally modern.
Es totalmente moderna.

Usually, the operation lasts only twenty minutes, the anesthetic doesn't hurt, and it is stitchless.
Usualmente, la operación solamente dura veinte minutos, el anestésico no duele y es sin suturas.

You'll be able to return home the same day.
Usted puede regresar a casa el mismo día.

Don't worry.
No se preocupe.

Let's make an appointment with the surgeon.
Vamos a hacer una cita con el cirujano.

Complications are rare.
Las complicaciones son raras.

In the majority of cases, much vision is regained.
En la mayoría de los casos, se recupera gran parte de la visión.

POSTERIOR CAPSULAR OPACIFICATION AND ND: YAG CAPSULOTOMY
OPACIFICACIÓN CAPSULAR POSTERIOR Y CAPSULOTOMÍA POR ND: YAG

You have an opacity of the membrane behind the lens implant.
Tiene una opacidad de la membrana detrás del lente implantado.

This is a common change one sees after cataract surgery.
Es un cambio común que se ve después de la cirugía para las cataratas.

The treatment is easy with a laser that (disperses/cleans/gets rid of) the opacity to restore good vision.
El tratamiento es fácil con un rayo láser que (desbarata/limpia/quita) la opacidad y restaura la buena visión.

After the laser removes the membrane opacity, it does not grow back.
Después que el láser remueve la opacidad de la membrana, la opacidad no vuelve a crecer.

GLAUCOMA
GLAUCOMA

Glaucoma is an eye disease.
El glaucoma es una enfermedad de los ojos.

One cannot cure it, but in most cases, one can control it.
No se puede curar, pero en la mayoría de los casos, se puede controlar.

Glaucoma is a disease that causes damage to the optic nerve.
El glaucoma es una enfermedad que causa daño al nervio óptico.

In many cases, the damage is due to high pressure in the eye.
En muchos de los casos, el daño se debe a alta presión en el ojo.

At other times, it's because there is a problem with blood circulation to the nerve.
Otras veces, es porque hay un problema con la circulación de sangre para el nervio.

This disease is dangerous because it can make you blind (m./f.), without showing any early symptoms.
Esta enfermedad es peligrosa porque le puede dejar ciego/a, sin mostrar síntomas al comienzo.

It doesn't hurt, and it affects the peripheral vision first.
No duele y afecta la visión periférica primero.

It is very important that you always use the drops to control it and have frequent eye (exams/checkups) as indicated by your doctor.
Es muy importante que usted siempre use las gotas para controlarla y que tenga (exámenes/chequeos) de los ojos frecuentes según le indique su doctor.

DIABETIC RETINOPATHY
RETINOPATÍA DIABÉTICA

All patients with diabetes must have a yearly dilated eye exam to prevent serious complications.
Todos los pacientes con diabetes deben tener un examen de ojo dilatado cada año para prevenir complicaciones serias.

If the blood sugar level is too high for an extended period of time, the blood vessels in the eye and rest of the body can leak and result in problems.
Si el nivel de azúcar en la sangre es muy alto por un periodo extendido de tiempo, los vasos sanguíneos en el ojo y en el resto del cuerpo pueden gotear y resultar en problemas.

You need to make an appointment with a specialist for a study of the blood vessels in the eye, and perhaps laser treatment.
Usted debe hacer una cita con un/a especialista para un estudio de los vasos sanguíneos en el ojo, y tal vez, un tratamiento con rayo láser.

The blood vessels inside the eye are (bleeding/leaking fluid).
Los vasos sanguíneos dentro del ojo están (sangrando/ goteando fluido).

This indicates that the blood sugar level is poorly controlled.
Esto indica que el nivel de azúcar en la sangre está mal controlado.

It is important to maintain the blood sugar at a correct and constant level because if not, you will have serious problems with your entire body.
Es importante mantener el azúcar en la sangre en un nivel correcto y constante porque si no, va a tener problemas serios en todo su cuerpo.

Diabetes affects all the blood vessels—not just in the eyes, but also in the heart, the legs, arms, kidneys, and brain.
La diabetes afecta a todos los vasos sanguíneos—no solamente a los de los ojos sino también a los del corazón, las piernas, los brazos, los riñones y el cerebro.

RETINAL LATTICE AND HOLES
ADELGAZAMIENTO Y AGUJEROS DE LA RETINA

Some parts of your retina are thin and weak.
Algunas partes de su retina están delgadas y débiles.

A possible occurrence is that the retina can detach.
Lo que puede pasar es que se desprenda la retina.

This is somewhat rare, but the probability is a little higher than among the general population.
Esto es un poco raro que suceda, pero la probabilidad es un poco mayor que en la población en general.

You need to (return/come) each year for an exam with pupil dilation.
Usted debe (regresar/volver) cada año para un examen con dilatación de la pupila.

If you suddenly see little lights or spots, you need to attend to it as soon as possible.
Si usted de repente ve lucecitas o manchas, debe atenderse lo más pronto posible.

Sometimes these symptoms indicate a problem with the retina.
A veces tales síntomas significan que hay un problema en la retina.

Chapter 23
Office Administration

Capítulo 23
Administración de la Oficina

ANSWERING THE PHONE
CONTESTAR EL TELÉFONO

Patient: **Do you speak Spanish?**
¿Usted habla español?

Staff: **I speak a little Spanish. I will try my best to help you. If necessary, I will get my coworker, Rosa, to help. She speaks Spanish.**
Yo hablo un poco de español. Voy a tratar de ayudarle. Si es necesario, buscaré a mi compañera, Rosa, para que me ayude. Ella habla español.

Staff: **I do not speak Spanish well. However, our doctor routinely performs exams in Spanish. If you have friends or family members that speak English, I can speak with one of them to schedule you an appointment with Dr. Smith.**
Yo no hablo español bien. Sin embargo, nuestro doctor hace exámenes en español de rutina. Si usted tiene amigos o familiares que hablan inglés, yo puedo hablar con uno de ellos para hacerle una cita con el Dr. Smith.

Staff: **Thank you for calling Dr. Smith's office. This is María. May I have your name?**
Gracias por llamar la oficina del Dr. Smith. Habla María. ¿Cómo se llama?

Patient: **Oscar Chávez.**
Oscar Chávez.

Staff: **Mr. Chávez, how may I help you?**
Sr. Chávez, ¿cómo puedo ayudarle?

DIRECTIONS TO THE OFFICE
DIRECCIONES A LA OFICINA

Our office is located at 9320 Carmel Mountain Road, Suite E. Driving from Highway 56, you'll want to exit onto Black Mountain Road and go north for three blocks. At Carmel Mountain Road, pass through the intersection and turn right into the first driveway. Our office is in a professional park. It is close to the high school.
Nuestra oficina está ubicada en 9320 Calle Carmel Mountain, Suite E. Manejando por el Highway 56, usted se va a salirse en la Calle Black Mountain y siga hacia el norte por tres cuadras. En la Calle Carmel Mountain, pase por la intersección y vire a la derecha en la primera entrada. Nuestra oficina está en un parque profesional. Está cerca de la escuela superior.

OFFICE HOURS
HORAS DE OFICINA

Our hours are eight to one and two to six, Monday through Friday.
Nuestras horas son de ocho a una y de dos a seis, de lunes a viernes.

Is there something I can help you with?
¿Hay algo con que puedo ayudarle?

POTENTIAL PATIENT INQUIRY
PREGUNTAS POSIBLES DEL PACIENTE

Patient: **I am interested in having an eye exam. How much does an eye examination cost?**
Estoy interesado/a en tener un examen de la vista. ¿Cuánto cuesta un examen de la vista?

Staff: **Thank you for asking. Our comprehensive eye examination includes a thorough evaluation of the internal and external eye health to rule out diseases** like cataracts, glaucoma, and macular degeneration. We use the latest in diagnostic instruments to measure eye pressure, color vision, depth perception, eye muscle coordination, and side vision and to evaluate for glasses. The cost of our comprehensive eye examination is $150.

Gracias por preguntar. Nuestro examen comprensivo incluye una evaluación minuciosa de la salud interna y externa del ojo para descartar las enfermedades como las cataratas, el glaucoma y la degeneración macular. Nosotros usamos los instrumentos de diagnósticos más modernos para medir la presión del ojo, la visión de color, la percepción de profundidad, la coordinación muscular del ojo y la visión lateral y para evaluar para anteojos. El costo de nuestro examen comprensivo es de $150.

VISION BENEFIT AND INSURANCE PLAN INQUIRIES
PREGUNTAS DE BENEFICIOS Y PLANES DE SEGUROS DE VISIÓN

Patient: **What vision plans do you accept?**
¿Qué seguros de visión ustedes aceptan?

Staff: **We accept all major vision plans that allow us to provide you with a high level of patient care.**
Nosotros aceptamos todos los seguros de visión principales que nos permiten proveerle con un alto nivel de cuidado de paciente.

Patient: **Do you accept Really Bad Vision Plan (RBVP)?**
¿Ustedes aceptan el Plan de Visión Muy Malo (PVBM)?

Staff: **Unfortunately, we don't accept your vision plan. You are still welcome to have your examination and purchase eyewear in our office—many of our patients choose to. But in such cases, you would be responsible for all fees.**
Desafortunadamente, no aceptamos su plan de visión. Usted está bienvenido a tener su examen y comprar sus anteojos en nuestra oficina—muchos de nuestros pacientes escogen hacerlo.

Pero en tal caso, usted sería responsable por todos los honorarios.

Patient: **Do you accept ABC medical insurance?**
¿Ustedes aceptan el seguro médico ABC?

Staff: **No, we are not an ABC medical insurance provider. Our office has unsuccessfully tried to become an ABC provider but ABC claims that they have enough providers. Please let your human resources department know that you would like to come to our office, but ABC medical insurance will not let us join their provider panel.**
No, no aceptamos el proveedor de seguro médico ABC. Nuestra oficina ha intentado sin éxito el convertirse en un proveedor de ABC pero ABC reclama que ya tienen suficientes proveedores. Por favor déjele saber a su departamento de recursos humanos que a usted le gustaría venir a nuestra oficina, pero el seguro médico ABC no nos permite unirnos a su panel de proveedores.

Patient: **What does my vision plan cover for professional services?**
¿Qué cubre mi plan de seguro de visión para servicios profesionales?

Staff: **Your plan covers the cost of your eye examination every 12 months with a $10 co-payment. You become exam-eligible this coming May 1. Your plan also provides you with a 15% savings on all contact lens services at any time.**
Su plan cubre el costo de su examen de la vista cada 12 meses con un co-pago de $10. Usted es elegible para el examen en mayo 1. Su plan también le provee con un descuento de 15% en todos los servicios de lentes de contacto en cualquier momento.

Patient: **What does my vision plan cover for glasses and contact lenses?**
¿Qué cubre mi plan de visión para anteojos y lentes de contacto?

Staff: **Your vision plan subsidizes the cost of glasses or contact lenses every 12 months, but not both at the same time. If you purchase glasses, you consume the benefits for contact lenses, and vice versa, for a 12-month period. If you need both glasses and contacts right now, we will apply your vision plan towards glasses to save you the most money.**

Su plan de visión subsidia el costo de los anteojos o lentes de contacto cada 12 meses, pero no a la misma vez. Si usted compra anteojos, usted consume sus beneficios para lentes de contacto y vice versa, por un periodo de 12 meses. Si usted necesita anteojos y lentes de contacto ahora, aplicaremos su plan de visión hacia el costo de sus anteojos para ahorrarle la mayor cantidad de dinero.

Patient: **More specifically, what does my vision plan cover for glasses?**

Más específicamente, ¿qué cubre mi plan de visión para los anteojos?

Staff: **Your vision plan provides you with a $150 allowance toward new frames every 24 months, and new standard lenses every 12 months. You have a $15 co-payment each time you order new glasses. Most of our patients choose to have premium lenses, like the thinner and lighter glare-free lenses. With your vision plan, you receive a special savings on them.**

Su plan de visión le provee con una asignación de $150 para aros nuevos cada 24 meses y lentes nuevos estándares cada 12 meses. Usted tiene un co-pago de $15 cada vez que ordena anteojos nuevos. La mayoría de nuestros pacientes escogen los lentes superiores, como los lentes más finos, más liviano y libres de reflejo. Con su plan de visión, usted recibe un descuento especial en éstos.

Staff: **This year, your vision plan provides you with a 20% savings on glasses. Your full allowance for new frames and lenses goes into effect next year.**

Este año, su plan de visión le provee un descuento de 20% en anteojos. Su asignación completa para los lentes y aros nuevos entra en efecto el próximo año.

Patient: **More specifically, what does my vision plan cover for contact lenses?**
Más específicamente, ¿qué cubre mi plan de visión para los lentes de contacto?

Staff: **Your plan gives you an allowance of $105 toward contact lenses every 12 months with a $15 co-payment. Since the allowance won't cover the entire annual cost of your contact lenses, you are responsible for the difference.**
Su plan de visión le provee con una asignación de $105 para los lentes de contacto cada 12 meses con un co-pago de $15. Como la asignación no cubrirá el costo anual completo de sus lentes de contacto, usted es responsable por la diferencia.

Staff: **Your vision plan covers a comprehensive eye health examination which includes the determination of the glasses prescription. It does not cover the cost of contact lenses or contact lens services due to their elective nature.**
Su plan de visión cubre un examen comprensivo de la salud de sus ojos lo cual incluye la determinación de la receta para anteojos. No cubre el costo de los lentes de contacto o los servicios de lentes de contacto debido a su naturaleza electiva.

Patient: **How much does it cost to get contact lenses?**
¿Cuánto cuesta el obtener lentes de contacto?

Staff: **Do you currently wear contact lenses?**
¿Usted usa lentes de contacto actualmente?

Staff: **If you do not currently wear contact lenses, you first need a comprehensive eye health examination. During that time, Dr. Smith will assess your need for corrective lenses. If you are a good candidate for contact lens wear, he will tell you what type would work best for you; for example, soft or rigid, disposable, astigmatism-correcting, multifocal, etc. Without knowing what type of contact lens is most appropriate for you, I cannot give you a specific fee quotation. But typical fees for new contact lens prescribing ranges from $148 for simple cases, to well** over $700 for complex situations, such as after corneal transplantation. Contact lenses themselves range from less than a dollar a pair for daily-disposable lenses, to over $100 for specialty lenses for extreme corrections.

Si usted no usa lentes de contacto actualmente, primero necesita un examen compresivo de la salud de sus ojos. Durante este tiempo, el Dr. Smith evaluará su necesidad de lentes correctivos. Si usted es un bien candidato para el uso de lentes de contacto, él le dirá qué tipo funcionará mejor para usted; por ejemplo, blandos o rígidos, desechables, correctores para astigmatismo, multifocales, etc. Sin saber qué tipo de lentes de contacto es más apropiado para usted, no puedo darle una cotización específica. Pero los honorarios típicos para la prescripción de lentes de contacto varían de $148 para casos simples, hasta más de $700 para situaciones complejas, tales como transplantes de córnea. Los lentes de contactos mismos varían de menos de un dólar para un par de lentes diarios desechables, hasta más de $100 para lentes especiales para correcciones extremas.

Patient: I already wear contact lenses but I am about to run out. So I need new contact lenses. How much will it cost?

Ya yo uso lentes de contacto pero se me están acabando. Así que necesito lentes de contacto nuevos. ¿Cuánto costará?

Staff: During your comprehensive eye examination, the doctor will also perform measurements to evaluate whether your existing contact lenses are best suited for your optimal vision, comfort, and eye health. When this contact lens service is done at the time of the examination, you are responsible for a $37 fee in addition to the fees for a comprehensive eye examination. In most cases, when no drastic changes in the lens design are necessary, the doctor can provide your contact lens prescription to fill afterwards. But if progress visits are necessary to finalize the contact lens prescription, additional fees apply for the additional time required.

Durante su examen de la vista compresivo, el doctor también tomará unas medidas para evaluar si sus lentes de contacto existentes son los mejores para su visión, comodidad y salud ocular óptima. Cuando se hace este servicio de lentes de contacto a la hora del examen, usted es responsable por el honorario de $37 adicional a los honorarios del examen de la vista comprensivo. En la mayoría de los casos, cuando no son necesarios cambios drásticos en el diseño del lente, el doctor puede darle su receta para lentes de contacto para que pueda comprarla. Pero si son necesarias visitas de progreso para finalizar la receta de lentes de contacto, honorarios adicionales aplican por el tiempo adicional requerido.

NEW PATIENT APPOINTMENT SCHEDULING
HACER CITAS PARA PACIENTES NUEVOS

Staff: **May I schedule an appointment for you?**
¿Puedo hacerle una cita?

Patient: **No, not at this time. Let me check my schedule and call back when I am ready.**
No, en este momento no. Déjeme verificar mi itinerario y le llamo para atrás cuando esté listo/a.

Staff: **Certainly. Meanwhile, you are welcome to learn more about our practice and services by visiting our website at www.YourTownOptometry.com. We look forward to hearing from you. Thank you for calling.**
Por supuesto. Mientras tanto, esta bienvenido/a a conocer más de nuestra práctica y nuestros servicios visitando nuestro sitio web en www.YourTownOptometry.com. Esperamos escuchar de usted otra vez. Gracias por llamar.

Patient: **Yes, I am ready to schedule an appointment.**
Sí, estoy listo para hacer una cita.

Staff: **Mr. Chávez, I have an appointment available with Dr. Smith for this Thursday at 1:00 p.m.**
Sr. Chávez, tengo una cita disponible con el Dr. Smith para este jueves a la 1:00 p.m.

Patient: **Yes, I would like that appointment.**
Sí, quisiera esa cita.

Patient: **That time does not work.**
Esa hora no funciona.

Staff: **Are there certain days of the week or times that seem to work best for you?**
¿Hay ciertos días de la semana u horas que parecen ser mejores para usted?

Patient: **Yes, I have Friday mornings off from work.**
Sí, yo tengo los viernes libres del trabajo.

Staff: **How about next Friday at 9:40 a.m.?**
¿Qué tal el próximo viernes a las 9:40 a.m.?

Patient: **Perfect.**
Perfecto.

Staff: **Excellent, Mr. Chávez. I think you'll enjoy your experience in our office. There are a few things I'll need in preparation for your exam. First, will you please confirm the spelling of your name?**
Excelente, Sr. Chávez. Creo que va a disfrutar su experiencia en nuestra oficina. Hay varias cosas que necesito para preparar su examen. Primero, ¿podría confirmar la ortografía de su nombre?

Staff: **I would like to save you time by mailing you our "welcome to the office" form. You can fill it out at your convenience and bring it to your appointment. What is your mailing address? You should receive the form along with our office brochure within two days. I also need your phone number where you can be reached in the unforeseen event there are changes.**
Me gustaría ahorrarle tiempo enviándole por correo nuestro formulario de "bienvenido a nuestra oficina". Usted puede llenarlo a su conveniencia y traerlo a su cita. ¿Cuál es su dirección postal? Usted debería recibir el formulario junto con el folleto de nuestra oficina dentro de dos días. También voy a necesitar su número de teléfono donde puedo conseguirlo en caso imprevisto que hayan cambios.

Staff: In order to save you time, I would encourage you to visit our office website at www.YourWebsite.com and download our "welcome to the office" form and complete it before your appointment tomorrow. On the website, you can also learn more about our services and get driving directions to our office.

Para ahorrarle tiempo, quisiera animarle a que visite el sitio web de nuestra oficina en www.YourWebsite.com y descargue nuestro formulario de "bienvenido a nuestra oficina" y lo complete antes de su cita mañana. En el sitio web, también puede aprender más acerca de los servicios que ofrecemos y obtener direcciones a nuestra oficina.

Staff: Since our examination is detailed, please allow yourself at least one hour. This should give you adequate time to select any eyewear as well.

Como su examen es detallado, por favor permítase por lo menos una hora. Esto debería darle tiempo adecuado para escoger los anteojos también.

ESTABLISHED PATIENT SCHEDULING EXAM
HACER CITAS PARA UN PACIENTE ESTABLECIDO

Patient: I would like to make an appointment with Dr. Smith.

Quisiera hacer una cita con el Dr. Smith.

Staff: Have you been in our office before?

¿Usted ha estado en nuestra oficina antes?

Patient: Yes, I got a reminder in the mail saying that I am due for my annual eye exam.

Sí, recibí un recordatorio en el correo diciendo que es tiempo para mi examen de la vista anual.

Staff: Thank you for calling. I am happy to make an appointment for you. Let's see … I just had an opening come up tomorrow afternoon at 2:20 p.m. Does that work for you?

Gracias por llamar. Sería un placer hacerle una cita. Veamos … acabo de tener un espacio disponible para mañana en la tarde a las 2:20 p.m. ¿Eso funciona para usted?

Staff: **Please bring any old glasses or contact lenses with you to the exam.**

Por favor traiga consigo sus anteojos o lentes de contacto viejos a su examen.

Staff: **Can I make appointments for any other family members at this time?**

¿Puedo hacer citas para otros miembros de su familia en este momento?

Patient: **Yes, I would also like to make an appointment for my (grandson/granddaughter/son/daughter/ husband/wife/mother/father/grandmother/ grandfather).**

Sí, también quisiera hacer una cita para mi (nieto/nieta/hijo/hija/esposo/esposa/madre/padre/ abuela/abuelo).

Patient: **Do you have any evening or Saturday appointments?**

¿Ustedes tienen citas por las tardes o los sábados?

Staff: **Yes we do. But since they are high demand, they book up very early. My next evening appointment is in four weeks. Should I reserve that time for you?**

Sí tenemos. Pero como están en alta demanda, se llenan rápido. Mi próxima cita por la tarde es en cuatro semanas. ¿Quiere que reserve ese tiempo para usted?

Staff: **In the unexpected event you need to change your appointment, please give us 48 hours notice to avoid a "broken appointment" fee.**

En el evento inesperado que usted necesite cambiar su cita, por favor avísenos con 48 horas de anticipación para evitar un honorario por "cita cancelada".

Staff: **Please wear your contact lenses when you come for your eye examination.**

Por favor use sus lentes de contacto cuando venga para su examen de la vista.

CALLS REGARDING ORDER STATUS
LLAMADAS SOBRE EL ESTADO DE
UNA ORDEN

Patient: **Could you please check whether my glasses and contact lenses have come in?**

¿Podría verificar si mis anteojos y lentes de contacto han llegado?

Staff: **I would be happy to check. What is your last name? Thank you. Please give me a moment to check.**

Sería un placer verificar. ¿Cuál es su apellido? Gracias. Por favor déme un momento para verificar.

Staff: **Yes, your glasses have arrived and you may schedule an appointment so that a frame and lens specialist can dispense them.**

Sí, sus anteojos llegaron y usted puede hacer una cita para que un especialista de aros y lentes los dispense.

Staff: **Your glasses are expected to arrive by next Tuesday because the lenses are back-ordered.**

Se espera que sus anteojos lleguen el próximo martes porque los lentes están atrasados.

Staff: **This message is for Mr. Cabrera. This is María from Dr. Smith's office. I am calling to let you know that your glasses are now ready for dispensing. Please call our office at _____ to set up a time for one of our opticians to custom adjust the frames to your face and instruct you on their proper use and care.**

Este mensaje es para el Sr. Cabrera. Ésta es María de la oficina del Dr. Smith. Estoy llamando para dejarle saber que sus anteojos están listos para ser dispensados. Por favor llame a nuestra oficina al _____ para establecer una hora en que nuestro óptico puede ajustar los aros a su cara y enseñarle el cuidado y uso apropiado.

PATIENT WHO HAS PROBLEMS WITH NEW GLASSES
PACIENTE QUE TIENE PROBLEMAS CON LOS ANTEOJOS NUEVOS

Patient: **I am having problems with my new glasses. I cannot see well with them and they make me uncomfortable.**

Tengo problemas con mis anteojos nuevos. No puedo ver bien con ellos y me hacen sentir incómodo/a.

Staff: **Thank you for bringing this to my attention. I am concerned and would like you to come into the office. One of our staff will gladly verify that your glasses were made according to the doctor's prescription and that they are properly fitted. Can you make it into our office at 3:30 p.m. today?**

Gracias por traer esto a nuestra atención. Estoy preocupado/a y me gustaría que viniera a la oficina. Uno de los miembros de nuestro personal con gusto verificará que sus anteojos se hicieron según la receta del doctor y que están bien ajustados. ¿Podría venir a nuestra oficina a las 3:30 p.m. de hoy?

CANCELING AND RESCHEDULING PATIENTS
CANCELAR Y CAMBIAR CITAS DE PACIENTES

Patient: **My name is Sandra Martínez and I have an appointment today at 2:30 p.m. However I need to cancel the appointment because I am sick.**

Mi nombre es Sandra Martínez y tengo una cita para hoy a las 2:30 p.m. Sin embargo necesito cancelar la cita porque estoy enferma.

Staff: **Thank you for your courtesy. I am sorry to hear that you are sick. May I reschedule this appointment for you?**

Gracias por su cortesía. Lo siento que esté enferma. ¿Puedo cambiarle la cita?

Patient: **I will need to check my schedule and call back. Is that okay?**

Necesito verificar mi itinerario y llamaré nuevamente. ¿Está bien?

Staff: Yes. When you are ready to reschedule, please call our office. We look forward to seeing you.

Sí. Cuándo usted esté lista para cambiar su cita, por favor llame a la oficina. Esperamos verle.

REMINDER PHONE CALLS
LLAMADAS DE RECUERDO

Staff: This is María from Dr. Smith's office reminding Mr. Chávez of his eye appointment at 9:40 a.m. Please remember to bring any existing glasses or contact lenses, along with your completed registration form. We look forward to seeing you. Should you have any questions, please call _____.

Ésta es María de la oficina del Dr. Smith recordándole al Sr. Chávez de su cita a las 9:40 a.m. Por favor, acuérdese de traer cualquier par de anteojos o lentes de contacto existentes, junto con su formulario de registro completado. Esperamos verle. Si tiene alguna pregunta, por favor llame al

_____.

PATIENT HAS NOT SHOWN UP ON TIME
PACIENTE QUE NO LLEGÓ A TIEMPO

Staff: This is María from Dr. Smith's office. I'm calling because I'm concerned. You had reserved time with Dr. Smith for an eye examination at 10:15 a.m. Is everything okay?

Ésta es María de la oficina del Dr. Smith. Estoy llamando porque estoy preocupada. Usted tenía tiempo reservado con el Dr. Smith para un examen de la vista a las 10:15 a.m. ¿Está todo bien?

Patient: Oh no, I forgot! I am sorry.

¡Oh no, se me olvidó! Lo siento.

Staff: Everyone forgets things once in a while. I would be happy to reschedule an appointment for you with Dr. Smith. I just had an opening come up for tomorrow morning at 9:00 a.m. Can you make that time?

Todos olvidamos las cosas de vez en cuando. Sería un placer cambiarle su cita con el Dr. Smith. Acabo de tener un espacio disponible para mañana en la mañana a las 9:00 a.m. ¿Usted puede venir a esa hora?

Staff: **Is there anything else I can help you with today?**
¿Hay algo más con lo que puedo ayudarle?

Staff: **Thank you for calling Dr. Smith's office.**
Gracias por llamar a la oficina del Dr. Smith.

PATIENT WITH HISTORY OF NOT SHOWING UP
PACIENTE CON ANTECEDENTES DE AUSENCIAS

Staff: **Mr. Martínez, since you have missed your second appointment in a row I cannot pre-appoint you onto our schedule. However, I can put you on our priority appointment list for same-day appointments. If we have a last-minute examination arise, I would be happy to call you to let you know that you can come in. Would you like me to do that?**
Sr. Martínez, como usted faltó a su segunda cita corrida, yo no puedo hacerle una cita en nuestro itinerario. Sin embargo, puedo colocarlo en nuestra lista de citas de prioridad para citas del mismo día. Si tenemos un examen que se abre a última hora, sería un placer llamarlo para dejarle saber que puede venir. ¿Le gustaría hacer eso?

CALLER WHO WISHES TO SPEAK WITH THE DOCTOR
PERSONA QUE LLAMA Y DESEA HABLAR CON EL DOCTOR

Patient: **I would like to speak with Dr. Smith.**
Quisiera hablar con el Dr. Smith.

Staff: **Absolutely. What is your name?**
Absolutamente. ¿Cómo usted se llama?

Patient: **Roberta Domínguez.**
Roberta Domínguez.

Staff: **Can you confirm the spelling of your full name?**
¿Podría confirmar la ortografía de su nombre completo?

Staff: **What does your call regard?**
¿Con respecto a qué es su llamada?

Staff: **Is this something that I can help you with?**
¿Es esto algo con que puedo ayudarle?

Staff: **Dr. Smith is with a patient right now. Would you like me to put you into his voice mail?**
El Dr. Smith está con un paciente ahora mismo. ¿Le gustaría que lo conecte con su correo de voz?

Staff: **Dr. Smith is out of the office at a meeting until next week. Would you like me to take a message for him?**
El Dr. Smith está fuera de la oficina en una reunión hasta la próxima semana. ¿Le gustaría dejarle un mensaje?

Patient: **That's not necessary. I will try calling back again in one week.**
Eso no es necesario. Yo trataré de llamar otra vez en una semana.

CHECKING OUT AND COLLECTING FEES
DESPIDO Y COBRO DE HONORARIOS

Staff: **Your total today is $385.**
Su total para hoy es $385.

Staff: **Will you be paying with cash, check, or credit card?**
¿Va a pagar con (dinero/en efectivo), con cheque o con tarjeta de crédito?

Patient: **Can I pay for part of the bill today, and the remainder at the next visit?**
¿Puedo pagar por parte de la factura hoy y el resto en la próxima visita?

Staff: **We cannot order your glasses until they are paid for. If it is more convenient, you can pay for your examination today and I can hold off ordering your glasses until you are ready to pay for them. Would you like me to do that?**

Nosotros no podemos ordenar sus anteojos hasta que estén pagos. Si es más conveniente para usted, usted puede pagar por su examen hoy y yo puedo esperar para ordenar sus anteojos hasta que usted esté listo/a para pagar por ellos. ¿Le gustaría hacer eso?

Staff: **Will you please sign here indicating that you agree to the charges?**

¿Podría firmar aquí indicando que usted está de acuerdo con los cargos?

Staff: **Thank you very much. This receipt is for your records. You should receive a phone call when your order arrives.**

Muchas gracias. Este recibo es para sus archivos. Usted debería recibir una llamada cuando llegue su orden.

The fee for this procedure is fifty dollars.

Los honorarios para este procedimiento son cincuenta dólares.

The insurance (formal/informal) covers this.

(La aseguranza/El seguro) cubre esto.

You need to pay just the co-payment of ten dollars.

A usted le toca pagar sólo el co-pago que son diez dólares.

We need (a deposit/an advance payment) for the laboratory to start the work.

Necesitamos un (depósito/anticipo) para que el laboratorio comience el trabajo.

**An advance payment is required to start
the job.**
Se requiere un anticipo para comenzar el trabajo.

**An advance payment is requested to start
the job.**
Se pide un anticipo para comenzar el trabajo.

MAKING REFERRALS AND FUTURE
   APPOINTMENTS
HACIENDO REFERIDOS Y CITAS FUTURAS

**I'm going to refer you (m./f.) to a (specialist/general
doctor).**
(Lo/La) voy a referir con un (especialista/doctor general).

**After your visit with the specialist, continue seeing me
for your routine exams.**
Después de su visita con el/la especialista, continúe conmigo
para sus exámenes usuales.

**Let us make an appointment in (a week
from today/two weeks from today) so that
I can (reexamine/check up) the eyes. Is that
all right?**
Vamos a apuntarle una cita dentro de (una semana/dos
semanas) para que yo le vuelva a examinar (revisar) los ojos.
¿Está bien?

**We are going to make an appointment for another eye
exam in one week. Is that all right?**
Vamos a hacerle una cita para otro examen de los ojos en una
semana. ¿Está bien?

I want to see you (m./f.) again in two weeks.
Quiero (verlo/a) otra vez en dos semanas.

Don't skip the next visit. It is very important.
No falte a la próxima visita. Es muy importante.

Keep your medical appointments.
Acuda a las citas médicas.

**I will see you (m./f.) again in one year. But if you
(think/perceive/suspect) there is a problem with the
eyes, certainly, (return/respond) at once.**
(Lo/La) veré otra vez en un año. Pero si (piensa/le parece/
sospecha) que hay un problema con los ojos, claro,
(regrese/acuda) en seguida.

**Here is my (business) card with the telephone numbers
where you can call me.**
Aquí tiene mi tarjeta (de presentación) con los números de
teléfonos a dónde me puede llamar.

English-to-Spanish Terminology

Terminología de Inglés a Español

DAYS OF THE WEEK	LOS DÍAS DE LA SEMANA
Monday	lunes
Tuesday	martes
Wednesday	miércoles
Thursday	jueves
Friday	viernes
Saturday	sábado
Sunday	domingo

MONTHS	LOS MESES
January	enero
February	febrero
March	marzo
April	abril
May	mayo
June	junio
July	julio
August	agosto
September	septiembre
October	octubre
November	noviembre
December	diciembre

ORDINAL NUMBERS	NÚMEROS ORDINALES
first	primero/a
second	segundo/a
third	tercero/a
fourth	cuarto/a
fifth	quinto/a
sixth	sexto/a

seventh	séptimo/a
eighth	octavo/a
ninth	noveno/a
tenth	décimo/a

	CARDINAL NUMBERS	**NÚMEROS CARDINALES**
0	zero	cero
1	one	un, uno/a
2	two	dos
3	three	tres
4	four	cuatro
5	five	cinco
6	six	seis
7	seven	siete
8	eight	ocho
9	nine	nueve
10	ten	diez
11	eleven	once
12	twelve	doce
13	thirteen	trece
14	fourteen	catorce
15	fifteen	quince
16	sixteen	dieciséis
17	seventeen	diecisiete
18	eighteen	dieciocho
19	nineteen	diecinueve
20	twenty	veinte
21	twenty-one	veintiuno
22	twenty-two	veintidós
23	twenty-three	veintitrés
24	twenty-four	veinticuatro
25	twenty-five	veinticinco
26	twenty-six	veintiséis
27	twenty-seven	veintisiete
28	twenty-eight	veintiocho
29	twenty-nine	veintinueve
30	thirty	treinta
40	forty	cuarenta
50	fifty	cincuenta
60	sixty	sesenta

70	seventy	setenta
80	eighty	ochenta
90	ninety	noventa
100	one hundred	cien (ciento)
101	one hundred one	ciento uno
102	one hundred two	ciento dos
103	one hundred three	ciento tres
104	one hundred four	ciento cuatro
105	one hundred five	ciento cinco
106	one hundred six	ciento seis
107	one hundred seven	ciento siete
108	one hundred eight	ciento ocho
109	one hundred nine	ciento nueve
110	one hundred ten	ciento diez
200	two hundred	doscientos
300	three hundred	trescientos
400	four hundred	cuatrocientos
500	five hundred	quinientos
600	six hundred	seiscientos
700	seven hundred	setecientos
800	eight hundred	ochocientos
900	nine hundred	novecientos
1000	one thousand	mil
1991	one thousand nine hundred ninety-one	mil novecientos noventa y uno
2001	two thousand one	dos mil uno
2005	two thousand five	dos mil cinco
2006	two thousand six	dos mil seis
2007	two thousand seven	dos mil siete
2008	two thousand eight	dos mil ocho
2009	two thousand nine	dos mil nueve
2010	two thousand ten	dos mil diez

INTERROGATIVE*	PALABRAS INTERROGATIVAS
How?	¿Cómo?
How far?	¿A qué distancia?
How often?	¿Con qué frecuencia?
How much?	¿Cuánto?
How many?	¿Cuántos?

How long?	¿Cuánto tiempo?
How many times?	¿Cuántas veces?
What?	¿Qué?
What else?	¿Qué más?
What for?	¿Para qué?
When?	¿Cuándo?
Where?	¿Dónde?
From where?	¿De dónde?
To where?	¿Adónde?
Which?	¿Cuál?
Which (ones)?	¿Cuáles?
Who?	¿Quién?
To whom?	¿A quién?
Whose?	¿De quién?
Why?	¿Por qué?

EXPRESSIONS OF TIME* / EXPRESIONES DE TIEMPO

year	el año
month	el mes
week	la semana
day	el día
hour	la hora
minute	el minuto
second	el segundo
today	hoy
tomorrow	mañana
day after tomorrow	pasado mañana
yesterday	ayer
day before yesterday	anteayer
tonight	esta noche
last night	anoche
tomorrow morning	mañana por la mañana
tomorrow afternoon	mañana por la tarde
tomorrow evening	mañana por la noche
every morning	cada mañana, todas las mañanas
every afternoon	cada tarde, todas las tardes
every evening	todas las noches
every night	cada noche
in the morning	por la mañana

in the afternoon	por la tarde
in the evening	por la noche
at night	en la noche
all morning	toda la mañana
all afternoon	toda la tarde
all night	toda la noche
two days ago	hace dos días
three weeks ago	hace tres semanas
six years ago	hace seis años
always	siempre
never	nunca
sometimes	algunas veces, a veces
from time to time	de vez en cuando
now	ahora
right now	ahora mismo
before	antes
after	después
later	más tarde
next week	la semana próxima
next year	el año próximo
until	hasta

CLOTHING*   LA ROPA

bathing suit	el traje de baño
bathrobe	la bata (de baño)
belt	el cinturón
blouse	la blusa
bluejeans	los levis
boot	la bota
brassiere	el sostén, los portabustos
button	el botón
cap	la gorra
coat	el abrigo
collar	el cuello
corset	el corsé
diaper	el pañal
dress	el vestido
hat	el sombrero
heel	el tacón
low heels	los tacones bajos
high heels	los tacones altos

hose	las medias
hospital gown	el camisón
jacket	la chaqueta
light weight (light clothes)	ligero (la ropa ligera)
nightgown	el camisón de dormir
oxford shoes	los zapatos bajos
pajamas	las pijamas
panties	las pantaletas
pants	los pantalones
rubber pants	los pantalones de plástico
sandals	las sandalias
scarf	la bufanda
shirt	la camisa
undershirt	la camiseta
t-shirt	la camiseta
shoe	el zapato
shorts (men's)	los calzones, los pantalones cortos
skirt	la falda, la pollera
sleeve	la manga
long	larga
short	corta
slipper	la zapatilla, la chancleta
sneakers	los zapatos de goma
socks	los calcetines
stockings	las medias
suit	el traje
sweater	el suéter
tie	la corbata
trousers	los pantalones
underwear	la ropa interior
vest	el chaleco

FAMILY MEMBERS (RELATIVES)*

MIEMBROS DE LA FAMILIA (PARIENTES)

aunt	la tía
brother	el hermano
brother-in-law	el cuñado
children	los hijos, los niños
cousin	el (la) primo(a)
daughter	la hija

daughter-in-law	la nuera
father	el padre, el papá
father-in-law	el suegro
grandfather	el abuelo
grandmother	la abuela
husband	el esposo, el marido
in-laws	los suegros
mother	la madre, la mamá
mother-in-law	la suegra
nephew	el sobrino
niece	la sobrina
parents	los padres
sister	la hermana
sister-in-law	la cuñada
son	el hijo
son-in-law	el yerno
uncle	el tío
wife	la esposa, la mujer

TIME ON THE CLOCK
LA HORA

To tell time in Spanish, use the verb ser + la(s) and the number.

What time is it?
¿Qué hora es?

It is seven o'clock.
Son las siete.

It is one o'clock.
Es la una.

It is eight o'clock.
Son las ocho.

It is two o'clock.
Son las dos.

It is nine o'clock.
Son las nueve.

It is three o'clock.
Son las tres.

It is ten o'clock.
Son las diez.

It is four o'clock.
Son las cuatro.

It is eleven o'clock.
Son las once.

It is five o'clock.
Son las cinco.

It is twelve o'clock.
Son las doce.

It is six o'clock.
Son las seis.

Use "media" for "30" or half past the hour:

It is 3:30.
Son las tres y media.

A.M. = de la mañana

P.M. = de la tarde (from noon until 6 o'clock)

P.M. = de la noche (from 6 until midnight)

On the right side of the clock, use "y" when expressing minutes:

It is ten after one.
Es la una y diez.

It is two fifteen.
Son las dos y cuarto.

It is three fifteen.
Son las tres y quince.

It is three thirty.
Son las tres y media.

On the left side of the clock, use "menos" or "falta(n):"

It is twenty to two.
Son las dos menos veinte.

It is five to eight.
Son las ocho menos cinco.

It is twenty to two.
Faltan veinte para las dos.

It is five to eight.
Faltan cinco para las ocho.

TIME EXPRESSIONS
EXPRESIONES DE TIEMPO

At what time?
¿A qué hora?

At eight o'clock.
A las ocho.

At noon.
Al mediodía.

At midnight.
A la medianoche.

early
temprano

late
tarde

on time
a tiempo

COLORS

	LOS COLORES
black	negro/a
blue	azul
bluish	azulado/a
brown	café
clear, light (in color tone)	claro/a
dark	oscuro/a
gold	dorado/a
gray	gris
green	verde
orange	anaranjado/a
pale	pálido/a
pink	rosa
purple	púrpura, morado/a
red	rojo/a, colorado/a
reddish	rojizo/a
silver	plateado/a
transparent	transparente
white	blanco/a
yellow	amarillo/a
yellowish	amarillento/a

THE OFFICE

	LA OFICINA
administration	la administración
assistant	el/la asistente
bathroom	el baño, el servicio
cashier	el cajero
chair	la silla
entrance	la entrada
exam (room/room)	el (salón/cuarto) de examen
exam record	el expediente
exit	la salida
hallway	el pasillo
laboratory	el laboratorio
optical dispensary	la óptica
ophthalmic technician	el técnico oftálmico/la técnica oftálmica
ophthalmologist	el oftalmólogo/la oftalmóloga
optometrist	el/la optómetra
public phone	el teléfono público

receptionist	el/la receptionista
specialist	el/la especialista
waiting room	el salón de espera

GENERAL HEALTH / LA SALUD GENERAL

allergy	la alergia
arthritis	la artritis
blood sugar	el azúcar en la sangre
bruise	el moretón
cancer	el cáncer
cold	el catarro, el resfriado
contagious	contagioso/a
diabetes	la diabetes
fever	la fiebre
freckle	la peca
flu	la gripe
headache	el dolor de cabeza
heart problems	los problemas cardiacos
high blood pressure	la alta presión sanguínea
pregnant	embarazada, esperando familia, en estado
thyroid problems	los problemas de la tiroides
wart	la verruga

EYE DISEASES / ENFERMEDADES DEL OJO

abrasion	la abrasión
blindness	la ceguera
burn	la quemadura
cataract	la catarata
color blindness	el daltonismo
defect	el defecto
discharge	las lagañas
dry eye	el ojo reseco
glaucoma	el glaucoma
infection	la infección
inflammation	la inflamación
injury	la lesión
mucus	la mucosidad
pinguecula, pterygium	la pinguécula, el pterigión, la carnosidad

red eye	el ojo rojo
scar	la cicatriz
surgery	la cirugía
trauma	el trauma
wound	la herida

SYMPTOMS

SÍNTOMAS

blurry	borroso
burn	ardor
clear	claro
cloudy	nublado
congested	congestionado/a
distortion	la distorsión
dizzy	mareado/a
eye dryness	resequedad del ojo
fluctuate	fluctúan
gradual	gradual
irritation	la irritación
itch	la comezón
pain	el dolor
sensitive to light	sensible a la luz
sudden	de repente
swelling	la hinchazón
tired	cansado/a
watery eyes	los ojos lagrimosos

THE EYE

EL OJO

blood vessels	los vasos sanguíneos
cornea	la córnea
crystalline lens	el lente cristalino
eyeball	el globo del ojo
eyebrow	la ceja
eyelid	el párpado
iris	el iris
lashes	las pestañas
muscles	los músculos
optic nerve	el nervio óptico
pupil	las pupilas (la niña del ojo)
retina	la retina
sclera	la esclerótica

skin	la piel
tear glands	las glándulas lacrimales
tears	las lágrimas

MEDICATIONS — MEDICAMENTOS

antibiotic	el antibiótico
artificial tears	las lágrimas artificiales
capsules	las cápsulas
daily	diariamente
drops	las gotas
by mouth	por boca
ointment	la pomada
pharmacy	la farmacia
pills	las pastillas
shake well	agite bien
tablets	las tabletas

EYECARE TERMS — TÉRMINOS DEL CUIDADO OCULAR

glasses	los anteojos
bifocals	los bifocales
eyeglass case	el estuche para los lentes
frames	los aros
glass	el cristal
nosepad	las patas en la parte de la nariz
plastic	el plástico
power	el aumento
prescription	la receta
prism	el prisma
progressive	los lentes progresivos
screw	el tornillo
sunglasses	los lentes de sol
tint	el tinte
ultraviolet light	la luz ultravioleta

Spanish-to-English Terminology

Terminología de Español a Inglés

A

la abrasión	abrasion
el abrigo	coat
abril	April
la abuela	grandmother
el abuelo	grandfather
la administración	administration
¿adónde?	to where?
agite bien	shake well
agosto	August
ahora	now
ahora mismo	right now
a la medianoche	at midnight
a las ocho	at eight o'clock
la alergia	allergy
algunas veces	sometimes
al mediodía	at noon
la alta presión sanguínea	high blood pressure
amarillento	yellowish
amarillo/a	yellow
anaranjado/a	orange

el año	year
anoche	last night
el año próximo	next year
anteayer	day before yesterday
los anteojos	glasses
antes	before
el antibiótico	antibiotic
¿a qué distancia?	how far?
¿a qué hora?	at what time?
¿a quién?	to whom?
los aros	frames
la artritis	arthritis
el/la asistente	assistant
a tiempo	on time
el aumento	power
ayer	yesterday
el azúcar en la sangre	blood sugar
azul	blue
azulado	bluish

B

el baño	bathroom
la bata (de baño)	bathrobe
los bifocales	bifocals
blanco/a	white
la blusa	blouse
borroso/a	blurry
la bota	boot

| el botón | button |
| la bufanda | scarf |

C

cada mañana	every morning
cada noche	every night
cada tarde	every afternoon
café	brown
el cajero	cashier
los calcetines	socks
los calzones	shorts
la camisa	shirt
la camiseta	undershirt, t-shirt
el camisón	hospital gown
el camisón de dormir	nightgown
el cáncer	cancer
cansado/a	tired
las cápsulas	capsules
la carnosidad	pinguecula, pterygium
las catarata	cataract
el catarro	cold
catorce	fourteen
la ceguera	blindness
la ceja	eyebrow
cero	zero
el chaleco	vest
la chancleta	slipper
la chaqueta	jacket
la cicatriz	scar

cien	one hundred
ciento	one hundred
ciento cinco	one hundred five
ciento cuatro	one hundred four
ciento diez	one hundred ten
ciento dos	one hundred two
ciento nueve	one hundred nine
ciento ocho	one hundred eight
ciento seis	one hundred six
ciento siete	one hundred seven
ciento tres	one hundred three
ciento uno	one hundred one
cinco	five
cincuenta	fifty
el cinturón	belt
la cirugía	surgery
claro/a	clear, light (in color tone)
colorado	red
la comezón	itch
¿cómo?	how?
congestionado/a	congested
¿con qué frecuencia?	how often?
contagioso/a	contagious
la córnea	cornea
el corsé	corset
el cristal	glass
¿cuál?	which?
¿cuáles?	which (ones)?

¿cuándo?	when?
¿cuántas veces?	how many times?
¿cuánto?	how much?
¿cuántos?	how many?
¿cuánto tiempo?	how long?
cuarenta	forty
cuarto/a	fourth
cuatro	four
cuatrocientos	four hundred
el cuello	collar
la cuñada	sister-in-law
el cuñado	brother-in-law

D

el daltonismo	color blindness
décimo/a	tenth
¿de dónde?	from where?
el defecto	defect
de la mañana	A.M. (in the morning)
de la noche	P.M. (at night; *from 6 until midnight*)
de la tarde	P.M. (in the afternoon; *from noon until 6 o'clock*)
¿de quién?	whose?
de repente	suddenly
después	after
de vez en cuando	from time to time
el día	day
la diabetes	diabetes

día de la semana	day of the week
diariamente	daily
diciembre	December
diecinueve	nineteen
dieciocho	eighteen
dieciséis	sixteen
diecisiete	seventeen
diez	ten
la distorsión	distortion
doce	twelve
el dolor	pain
el dolor de cabeza	headache
domingo	Sunday
¿dónde?	where?
dorado/a	gold (in color tone)
dos	two
doscientos	two hundred
dos mil y uno	two thousand one
dos mil cinco	two thousand five
dos mil seis	two thousand six
dos mil siete	two thousand seven
dos mil ocho	two thousand eight
dos mil nueve	two thousand nine
dos mil diez	two thousand ten

E

embarazada	pregnant
enero	January

en estado	pregnant
la enfermedad	disease
las enfermedades del ojo	eye diseases
la entrada	entrance
la esclerótica	sclera
es la una	it is one o'clock
es la una y diez	it is ten after one
esperando familia	pregnant
la esposa	wife
el esposo	husband
esta noche	tonight
el estuche para los lentes	eyeglass case
el expediente	exam record

F

la falda	skirt
faltan cinco para las ocho	it is five to eight
faltan veinte para las dos	it is twenty to two
la farmacia	pharmacy
febrero	February
la fiebre	fever
fluctuar	to fluctuate

G

las glándulas lacrimales	tear glands
la glaucoma	glaucoma
el globo del ojo	eyeball
el golpe	trauma
la gorra	cap

las gotas	drops
gradual	gradual
la gripe	flu
gris	gray

H

hace dos días	two days ago
hace seis años	six years ago
hace tres semanas	three weeks ago
hasta	until
la herida	wound
la hermana	sister
el hermano	brother
la hija	daughter
el hijo	son
los hijos	children
la hora	hour
hoy	today

I

la infección	infection
la inflamación	inflammation
el iris	iris
la irritación	irritation

J

jueves	Thursday
julio	July
junio	June

L

el laboratorio	laboratory
las lagañas	discharge
las lágrimas	tears
las lágrimas artificiales	artificial tears
el lente cristalino	crystalline lens
los lentes de sol	sunglasses
los lentes progresivos	progressive lenses
la lesión	injury
los levis	bluejeans
ligero	light weight
lunes	Monday
la luz ultravioleta	ultraviolet

M

la madre	mother
la mamá	mother
mañana	tomorrow
mañana por la mañana	tomorrow morning
mañana por la noche	tomorrow evening
mañana por la tarde	tomorrow afternoon
la manga	sleeve
la manga corta	short sleeve
la manga larga	long sleeve
mareado/a	dizzy
el marido	husband
martes	Tuesday
marzo	March
más tarde	later

mayo	May
las medias	hose, socks, stockings
los medicamentos	medications
el mes	month
miércoles	Wednesday
mil	one thousand
mil novecientos noventa y uno	one thousand nine hundred ninety-one
el minuto	minute
morado/a	purple
el moretón	bruise
mucoso	mucus
la mujer	wife, woman
los músculos	muscles

N

negro/a	black (m./f.)
el nervio óptico	optic nerve
la niña del ojo	pupil
los niños	children
novecientos	nine hundred
noveno/a	ninth
noventa	ninety
noviembre	November
nublado	cloudy
la nuera	daughter-in-law
nueve	nine
el número	number
nunca	never

O

ochenta	eighty
ocho	eight
ochocientos	eight hundred
octavo/a	eighth
octubre	October
la oficina	office
el/la oftalmólogo/a	ophthalmologist
el ojo	eye
el ojo rojo	red eye
el ojo reseco	dry eye
los ojos lagrimosos	watery eyes
la resequedad del ojo	eye dryness
once	eleven
la óptica	optical dispensary
el/la optómetra	optometrist
oscuro/a	dark

P

el padre	father
los padres	parents
pálido/a	pale (in color tone)
el pañal	diaper
las pantaletas	panties
los pantalones	pants
los pantalones de plástico	rubber pants
el papá	father
¿para qué?	what for?
los parientes	relatives

el párpado	eyelid
pasado mañana	day after tomorrow
el pasillo	hallway
las pastillas	pills
las patas en la parte de la nariz	nosepad
la peca	freckle
las pestañas	eyelashes
la piel	skin
las pijamas	pajamas
la pinguécula	pinguecula
el plástico	plastic
plateado/a	silver (in color tone)
la pollera	skirt
la pomada	ointment
por boca	by mouth
por la mañana	in the morning
por la noche	in the evening
por la tarde	in the afternoon
¿por qué?	why?
los portabustos	brassiere
primero/a	first
el/la primo/a	cousin
el prisma	prism
los problemas cardíacos	heart problems
los problemas de la tiroides	thyroid problems
el pterigión	pterygium
la pupila	pupil
púrpura	purple

Q

¿qué?	what?
¿qué hora es?	what time is it?
la quemadura	burn
¿qué más?	what else?
¿quién?	who?
quince	fifteen
quinientos	five hundred
quinto/a	fifth

R

el/la recepcionista	receptionist
la receta	prescription
el resfriado	cold
la retina	retina
rojizo/a	reddish
rojo/a	red
la ropa	clothing
la ropa interior	underwear
la ropa ligera	lightweight clothes
rosa	pink

S

sábado	Saturday
la salida	exit
el (salón/cuarto) de examen	exam (room)
el salón de espera	waiting room
la salud	health
las sandalias	sandals

el segundo	second (of time)
segundo/a	second
seis	six
seiscientos	six hundred
la semana	week
la semana próxima	next week
sensible a la luz	sensitive to light
septiembre	September
séptimo/a	seventh
el servicio	bathroom
sesenta	sixty
setecientos	seven hundred
setenta	seventy
sexto/a	sixth
siempre	always
siete	seven
la silla	chair
los síntomas	symptoms
la sobrina	niece
el sobrino	nephew
el sombrero	hat
son las cinco	it is five o'clock
son las cuatro	it is four o'clock
son las diez	it is ten o'clock
son las doce	it is twelve o'clock
son las dos	it is two o'clock
son las dos menos veinte	it is twenty to two
son las dos y cuarto	it is two fifteen

son las nueve	it is nine o'clock
son las ocho	it is eight o'clock
son las ocho menos cinco	it is five to eight
son las once	it is eleven o'clock
son las seis	it is six o'clock
son las siete	it is seven o'clock
son las tres	it is three o'clock
son las tres y media	it is three thirty
son las tres y quince	it is three fifteen
el sostén	brassiere
la suegra	mother-in-law
el suegro	father-in-law
los suegros	in-laws
el suéter	sweater

T

las tabletas	tablets
el tacón	heel
los tacones altos	high heels
los tacones bajos	low heels
tarde	late
el técnico oftálmico	ophthalmic technician
el teléfono público	public phone
temprano	early
tercero/a	third
la tía	aunt
el tinte	tint
el tío	uncle
toda la mañana	all morning

toda la noche	all night
toda la tarde	all afternoon
todas las mañanas	every morning
todas las noches	every evening
todas las tardes	every afternoon
el tornillo	screw
el traje	suit
el traje de baño	bathing suit
transparente	transparent
trece	thirteen
treinta	thirty
tres	three
trescientos	three hundred

U

uno/a	one

V

los vasos sanguíneos	blood vessels
veinte	twenty
veinticinco	twenty-five
veinticuatro	twenty-four
veintidós	twenty-two
veintinueve	twenty-nine
veintiocho	twenty-eight
veintiséis	twenty-six
veintisiete	twenty-seven
veintitrés	twenty-three
veintiuno	twenty-one

verde	green
la verruga	wart
el vestido	dress
viernes	Friday

Y

el yerno	son-in-law

Z

la zapatilla	slipper
el zapato	shoe
los zapatos bajos	oxford shoes
los zapatos de goma	sneakers

Informal Expressions

Expressiones Informales

Really?

¿De veras?

Cool!

¡Qué chévere!

Awesome!

¡Qué padre!

My God!

¡Díos mío!

(All right then/Now what)?

¿Ahora pues?

All done (ready to move on)?

¿Ya estuvo?

You (don't/didn't) notice what happened?

¿No te (das/diste) cuenta?

Don't lose heart. (Don't give up.)

No te agites.

Index

Índice

A

Accommodation, near testing with relative, 44–45

Acuity
pinhole, 21–22
stereo, 28–29

Acuity, visual, 19–23
eye charts for illiterates, 22–23
measurement, 20–21
pinhole acuity, 21–22
preparation, 19–20

Adaptations, explaining, 67–69

Administration, office, 101–119
answering phone, 101–102
caller who wishes to speak with doctor, 115–116
calls regarding order status, 112
canceling and rescheduling patients, 113–114
checking out, 116–118
collecting fees, 116–118
directions to office, 102
establishing patient scheduling exam, 110–111
future appointments, 118–119
insurance plan inquiries, 103–108
making referrals, 118–119
new patient appointment scheduling, 108–110
office hours, 102
patients who have not shown up on time, 114–115
patients who have problems with new glasses, 113
patients with histories of not showing up, 115
potential patient inquiry, 102–103

Administration, office—cont'd
reminder phone calls, 114
vision benefits, 103–108

Advance payment for laboratory work, 117

Air, contamination in, 94

Allergic conjunctivitis, 92

Allergies, medications and, 18

Amblyopia, occlusion therapy for, 72–73

Amsler grid, 37–38

Anesthetic drops, 54

Anesthetize eyes, 58

Annual eye exam, 110

Answering phone, 101–102

Antibiotic drops, 58

Antireflective coating, 63

Antiscratch/antireflective coatings, 63

Appointment scheduling, new patient, 108–110

Appointments
change in, 111
evening, 111
future, 118–119
keeping medical, 119
rescheduling, 113–114
Saturday, 111

Artificial tears, 78, 92–94

Aspheric lenses, 64

Astigmatism, 80

Automated-Humphrey visual field, 36

B

Back-ordered lenses, 112

Back-up pair of glasses, 63

Bacteria on eyelids, 91

153

SYSTEM REQUIREMENTS
Intel Pentium II processor or higher
Tray-loading CD-ROM
Microsoft Windows 98, 2000, NT 4.0, ME, or XP
Monitor 800 × 600 screen resolution, 256 colors
Audio speakers and 16-bit 22-khz audio card (SoundBlaster
 compatible)
64 MB of available RAM

Supported Browsers: Internet Explorer 5.x, and Netscape 7.x.
 To download the most current version of Internet Explorer,
 please visit www.microsoft.com. To download the most
 current version of Netscape, please visit www.netscape.com.

Audio for *Spanish Terminology for the Eyecare Team* requires
 Quicktime 6.1 or higher. An internet connection is required
 when installing Quicktime from the CD.

INSTALLATION INSTRUCTIONS
After you place the CD into the CD-ROM drive, the CD will
 automatically load into your default browser.

If this does not occur, click Start and select Run. In the prompt,
 type "D:\start.html" where D is the letter of CD-ROM drive.
 Press OK to load *Spanish Terminology for the Eyecare Team*.

This product requires Quicktime 6.1 or higher to run properly.
 If you do not have this product installed, you may install
 Quicktime 6.1 from the CD. These installers are located in
 the quicktime_installers folder.

To download the most current version of Quicktime instead,
 please visit the following link to download a free version of
 Quicktime.
 http:www.apple.com/quicktime/download

How to change your default browser in Windows

Instructions on how to change your default browser are in the
documentation of your browser. Instructions for common
browsers follow.

Internet Explorer 6.0

1. Open Internet Explorer.
2. Select Tools/Internet Options.
3. Select the Programs tab.
4. Click the Reset Web Settings button.
5. Click Yes.
6. Close Internet Explorer.

Netscape

1. Open Netscape 7.1
2. If Netscape asks if you want to change your default
   browser select OK and close Netscape.
3. Otherwise, select Edit/Preferences.
4. Select the Navigator tab and click the Set Default Browser
   button.
5. Close Netscape.

TECHNICAL SUPPORT

Technical Support for this product is available between 7 AM
and 7 PM CST Monday through Friday. Before calling, be sure
that your computer meets the minimum system requirements
to run this software. Inside the United States and Canada,
call 1-800-692-9010. Outside North America,
call 314-872-8370. You may also fax your questions to
314-997-5080, or contact Technical Support through
e-mail: technical.support@elsevier.com.

Copyright © 2006 by Elsevier Inc.

Part Number: 9996007340